THE
FOOD
CONNECTION

THE FOOD CONNECTION

How the Things You Eat Affect the Way You Feel — And What You Can Do About It

David Sheinkin, M.D.;
Michael Schachter, M.D.;
and Richard Hutton

Introduction by Dr. Carlton Fredericks

THE BOBBS-MERRILL COMPANY, INC.
Indianapolis / New York

Published by The Bobbs-Merrill Company, Inc.
Indianapolis   New York
Designed by Rita Muncie
Manufactured in the United States of America

First printing

Library of Congress Cataloging in Publication Data

Sheinkin, David, 1939–
  The food connection.

  Bibliography: p.
  Includes index.
  1. Mental illness—Nutritional aspects.
2. Food allergy—Nutritional aspects. 3. Brain—
Diseases. 4. Food habits. I. Schachter,
Michael, 1941–, joint author. II. Hutton,
Richard, joint author. III. Title.
RC455.4.N8S48   616.8′9   78-11208
ISBN 0-672-52518-6

To April
whose illness helped pave the way
for our understanding of the food connection

Acknowledgments

So many people have contributed to our understanding of the concepts presented in this book that to name them all would be impossible. However, the following have been most influential either through our direct contact with them or through their writings: Theron Randolph, M.D.; Marshall Mandell, M.D.; William Philpott, M.D.; Henry Newbold, M.D.; Lawrence Dickey, M.D.; Abram Hoffer, M.D.; Allan Cott, M.D.; David Hawkins, M.D.; Linus Pauling, Ph.D.; Carl Pfeiffer, M.D., Ph.D.; Ben Feingold, M.D.; Joseph Miller, M.D.; William Crook, M.D.; Broda Barnes, M.D.; John Diamond, M.D.; Warren Levin, M.D.; Beatrice Trum Hunter; Paavo Airola, Ph.D.; George Goodheart, D.C.; and the late John Tintera, M.D., and Herbert Rinkel, M.D.

We are particularly indebted to our friend and colleague Dr. Carlton Fredericks for his assistance in opening our minds to the whole area of nutritional and preventive medicine and for his comments on the manuscript.

Susan Shaw prepared the entire section (Appendix IV) on food families and the rotation diets, including menus. She was aided by Chapter 10 of *Clinical Ecology* by Dr. Alsoph H. Corwin, "The Rotating Diet and Taxonomy," pp. 122–48.

Lynn Sheinkin and Marlene Brodsky helped in editing certain

sections of the book, and Diane Giddis's tireless reviewing and editing of the entire manuscript were invaluable.

We would also like to thank Annette Siegel for her help in the preparation of the manuscript.

But most of all we would like to thank our patients, who continuously teach us how to help them.

Michael B. Schachter, M.D.
David Sheinkin, M.D.

Authors' Note

All the case histories cited in this book are authentic; we have not resorted to the practice of using composites—histories drawn from several patients and distilled into one dramatic story to make a point. We have altered descriptions of our patients only to preserve their anonymity, and although we usually do see our patients separately, we have elected to use the general "we" instead of our own names on our own cases in order to tell the stories more simply.

We wish to emphasize that although this book contains much useful information regarding the diagnosis and treatment of brain sensitivities, the material is for educational purposes only and is not intended for use in diagnosing or treating any individual. Furthermore, it is best that all procedures described herein be carried out under medical supervision.

David Sheinkin, M.D.
Michael Schachter, M.D.

CONTENTS

xiii INTRODUCTION by Dr. Carlton Fredericks

  1 ONE: Brain Sensitivity and You

 18 TWO: Crackpot Theory or Established Fact?

 34 THREE: Fasting and Deliberate Food Testing

 53 FOUR: The Coca Pulse Test

 62 FIVE: Kinesiologic Testing

 73 SIX: Four Laboratory Tests

 92 SEVEN: Complications

104 EIGHT: Treatment

135 APPENDIX 1: Signs and Symptoms That May Indicate Sensitivity Reactions

139 APPENDIX 2: Food Families and the Rotation Diet

166 APPENDIX 3: Tests to Determine Predisposing Factors

169 APPENDIX 4: Sprouting Seeds

172 APPENDIX 5: The Kaiser-Permanente (K-P) or Feingold Diet

173 APPENDIX 6: Resource Organizations

179 NOTES

187 BIBLIOGRAPHY

199 INDEX

INTRODUCTION

Drs. Michael Schachter and David Sheinkin have here written a book which proposes—with all justification—to persuade you that something present in your food or environment can be responsible for many symptoms of both mind and body. The fact that they're right will, it is hoped, speed professional acceptance of the thesis, although the "medical lag" to which these physicians refer is seemingly inevitable. I applaud this text for the good reason that it will rescue some of its readers—perhaps you—from years of gratuitous suffering.

As I wrote in another text: "Whether the psychosis is gene-dictated, or the price of intolerable strain, or the direct result of a derangement of the exquisitely concatenated chemistries of the brain and the nervous system, in the end the mental sickness is a molecular disease, or it is not a disease at all." *The Food Connection* adds to that statement: "The 'molecular' disease may be a reaction to something in your environment—food, drug, automobile exhaust, pollutants in water or air—and the impact may produce depression, anxiety, indigestion, arthritic pains, insomnia, claustrophobia, or any of a thousand physical and mental symptoms which, in the absence of accurate diagnosis, may place you on the psychiatric couch, or make you the target of endless prescriptions for palliative drugs."

A good example is a family in which the mother was a paranoid schizophrenic. Her oldest child was hearing voices from the clouds, and her youngest boy received visits from his (deceased) grandfather, who appeared at night as a purple cloud in his bedroom. All three reverted to total normality when wheat was withdrawn from their diets.

This is brain sensitivity. Allergists may call it allergy, but the terminology is less important than the concept, which has not received the attention it deserves. Allergy (or sensitivity) affects every other organ and tissue in the body; why should the brain be exempt? It isn't; any allergic person can tell you that during an attack he is likely to be irritable, unduly fatigued or nervous, or to feel depersonalized. Unfortunately, attention has been directed primarily to the more obvious impacts of such sensitivity —eczema, asthma, hay fever, and hives. Few realized that the brain alone might be the primary target and that deranged behavior and bizarre symptoms might be the result.

Sensitivity to the nightshade plants (such common foods as tomato, white potato and eggplant) can cause depression and, not incidentally, symptoms of a full-blown arthritis. A chlorine allergy can, for the sensitive, make a glass of water an invitation to anxiety, fear and trembling. A wheat sensitivity can trigger fits of weeping for which there is no explanation in the life situation. The wrong food can touch off a drop in the blood sugar, which in turn can cause claustrophobia. Hydrocarbon sensitivity can make plastic kitchen tiling the source of a feeling of unbearable apprehension. Submitted to a whiff of an aerosol spray of a disinfectant, a child removed light bulbs from ceiling fixtures and dropped them into a wastebasket, explaining that she was planting seeds in her garden. Her school accused her of using drugs. A physician versed in bioecologic allergy reproduced her symptoms by exposing her to the spray, which had been used in the school rest room.

The irony in this medical discovery comes when the patient discovers that he is addicted to the very foods which are his undoing, and that his symptoms are relieved by a dose of two vitamins or a dilution of the offending food. That is part of what you will learn in The Food Connection.

In our polluted world we are bombarded with substances nature never anticipated, and filled with foods that are vehicles for the alien and the unpredictable. Some of us walk like gods, unwounded all the way. Some of us land on psychiatric couches, when we should be visiting bioecological physicians. Some of us are plied with tranquilizers, antidepressants, or antihistamines, when we need a diet stripped of the substances that offend our brains. In *The Food Connection* Drs. Schachter and Sheinkin offer you an invaluable guide to preservation of sanity and good health. As past president of the International Academy of Preventive Medicine, I salute their contribution to prophylaxis.

Carlton Fredericks, Ph.D., F.I.A.P.M.

THE
FOOD
CONNECTION

ONE:
Brain Sensitivity and You

Many of you are suffering from a brain sensitivity, and neither you nor your doctor knows it. You might be complaining of symptoms ranging from occasional fatigue, irritability or headaches to chronic listlessness, anxiety and depression. All of these symptoms, and more, can be caused by a reaction of your brain to the foods you are eating.

Brain sensitivity exists on a scale that affects almost all of us, whether we are sufferers ourselves or are close to someone who is suffering. It affects millions who have been attributing their feelings of being rundown, irritable, or tired to "just one of those things," as well as those who have complained to their doctors about feeling not quite normal and who have been told in return, "It's all in your head."

Ironically, for many people their doctors are telling them at least part of the truth: their problems *are* in their heads. But they are physical, not just emotional or psychological; and their solutions may be much closer than years of therapy, tranquilizers, a regimen of vitamin pills, or a needed vacation. Help may, in fact, be as close as the tips of their tongues. For brain sensitivity *can* be diagnosed and treated.

Unfortunately, few physicians understand what brain sensitivity is, and even fewer know how to treat it. As a result, many of us are under the impression that the physical and psychological burdens we are carrying are an integral part of our lives. Even if we should decide to seek help, chances are that the doctor we consult won't even be aware that such a thing as brain sensitivity exists.

THE COOKIE MONSTER AND THE MILKMAN

The most recent such case that came to our attention is a clear example of this phenomenon. Mr. A is a bright and articulate fifty-eight-year-old architect. For thirty years he was tortured by recurring nightmares. He described the dreams as being so horrible that he was literally terrified to go to sleep; he would force himself to stay up as late as he could, and would only fall asleep when exhaustion took over. Within an hour or two of falling asleep he would wake up again, panicked by one of his nightmares. This pattern recurred each time he slept. In addition, for the same thirty-year period Mr. A had been suffering from severe and almost constant headaches. Also overweight, he attributed his obesity to overeating, which he felt he could not control. He was particularly tempted by cookies which he gulped down with the fervor of an addict. They were a major solace to him; he generally felt better after each cookie binge.

Mr. A had consulted many physicians, including a number of psychiatrists, and had tried many treatments, none of which brought him relief. He had been in psychotherapy with one of these psychiatrists for five years and felt that it had helped him to learn much, both about himself and about his nightmares; but despite all this valuable insight, the terrible dreams continued. For the preceding two years he had been treated by a highly regarded psychiatrist in the field of psychopharmacology (use of medication for the treatment of psychiatric conditions) who had access not only to routine psychiatric drugs but to the latest experimental drugs as well. During this period he had tried many different drugs, but only one seemed to decrease the intensity of his nightmares. After a few months, however, even that medication lost its effect, and the nightmares resumed their full intensity. Further efforts with medication failed, and it was at this point that Mr. A came to see us.

We had learned a good deal about brain sensitivity by then; we recognized its hallmarks almost immediately and pinpointed Mr. A's prime addiction—cookies—as one of the major sensitizing agents. He listened carefully and very skeptically as we explained the concept of brain sensitivity and outlined for him a plan of diagnosis and treatment. Because he was desperate, he agreed to go along with our recommendations. Within two weeks of beginning our program, his own experience convinced him that brain sensitivity can be a potent factor. He was suddenly completely free of the symptoms that had plagued him for more than half his life. For the first time in thirty years, he was able to sleep for six to eight hours a night; he had no nightmares; and he was no longer tormented by headaches.

To Mr. A the whole thing seemed somewhat miraculous. Even though we have now seen hundreds of cases of brain sensitivity, we still feel a sense of awe each time we see the results of this treatment. In fact, our success in our very first encounter with this condition, over five years ago, was just as dramatic.

When Mr. B, a chemist in his mid-forties, first consulted us, brain sensitivity was a term with which we were only vaguely familiar. Mr. B came to us feeling extremely depressed. He told us that he had been living in a state of depression for the past seventeen years, during which time he had attempted suicide at least three times. He described the onset of his problems as having come about quite suddenly. He was working at an industrial plant and was about to deliver a short report at a staff meeting. Just before he got up to speak, he experienced, without warning, an attack of anxiety. It was something that had never happened to him before. The fact that there was nothing unusual about the staff meeting and that he had routinely presented reports at those meetings in the past made his problem seem even more strange.

That episode was the first of a series of similar attacks; the feelings would appear suddenly, without explanation. Soon after, he had fallen into deep depression and had been seeking help ever since.

Mr. B had been in psychotherapy for many of those seventeen years. In addition, a few years after the appearance of his initial symptoms, he had undergone dozens of physical tests. His doctors found that he had hypoglycemia (low blood sugar) and advised him to undertake a high-protein, low-carbohydrate diet which included as much as a quart of milk a day. They also suggested that he suck on Lifesavers, since they would provide him with a quick dose of sugar to bolster his own level of blood sugar. (In our experience, eating Lifesavers—or any other food containing refined sugar—to alleviate low blood sugar symptoms generally makes the condition worse in the long run.)

When he drank a lot of milk and ate Lifesavers, his depression lifted slightly; but he was never completely free of it during those seventeen years. Sometimes it improved; sometimes it worsened. Sometimes he could work; sometimes he could not. Over the years, he developed a characteristic pattern of behavior: He would find a job and work well for a while; then the quality of his work would deteriorate. At that point he would resign (while he could still get a decent letter of recommendation) and begin anew at another job. He came to see us because he had recently moved again and needed a local psychiatrist who could continue what the others had begun.

We decided to put Mr. B on a program of orthomolecular treatment which we had added to our classical psychiatric training a year earlier. Orthomolecular (correct molecules) psychiatry deals with psychiatric conditions that stem from an imbalance in body chemistry, particularly from poor or improper nutrition. Treatment of many problems that seem to have psychological roots sometimes consists of simply adding missing nutrients to a patient's diet. We had found that the condition of many of our patients improved after their vitamin and mineral balances were corrected. Some patients improved without further need of psychotherapy; others became more responsive to traditional psychotherapy.

In the case of Mr. B, our tests confirmed the earlier diagnosis of hypoglycemia and indicated some mineral imbalances as well. We were optimistic that with proper attention to both the mineral imbalances and the hypoglycemia (our approach to hypoglycemia was considerably different from the treatment he was on), he would start to improve. But even though Mr. B stuck to the treatment program religiously, he failed to show any improvement. We tried varying the treatment in a number of ways, but nothing seemed to relieve his basic depression.

We didn't think of brain sensitivity until we had exhausted all other possibilities. Then we remembered having heard, at a psychiatric conference, about some cases in which psychiatric symptoms resulted from patients who were sensitive to certain foods. We explained the concepts as we understood them, pointing out to Mr. B that we had not as yet used them with other patients.

At that time, the only way we knew of to determine whether or not a food sensitivity existed was to fast (to abstain from all foods except water) for a minimum of four days and then to eat individual foods to see which, if any, produced symptoms. It didn't seem like a very promising approach, but seventeen years of depression had pushed Mr. B to the point of desperation. So, after appropriate consultation, we carefully devised a medically supervised fast for him.

On the first day of the fast, he experienced no change; on the second, his depression worsened; but on the third day, he reported that the depression was clearly lifting and that he was feeling better than before the fast. When he spoke to us on the fourth day, his voice was filled with excitement. His depression had left without a trace. He couldn't remember having felt so happy in over twenty years. We all had trouble believing it.

Mr. B remained free of depression for a few days, while we carefully reintroduced foods into his diet one at a time. Then, an hour after drinking milk, his old symptoms returned. "It was as if I were standing in a sunlit room, and suddenly someone pulled the shades down and everything got dark again," he said later. Fortunately, this bout with his old symptoms lasted only a few hours. Thereafter, he remained free of depression as long as he avoided milk and milk products. He went on to lead a normal life; and we, as professionals, had become a little wiser.

In the years between our treating Mr. A and Mr. B, we have been able to help hundreds of other people suffering from brain sensitivities. While the "cookie monster" and the "milkman" are two of our more dramatic cases, they are by no means isolated examples. However, figures reflecting the incidence of brain sensitivity in the population are hard to come by, because few physicians recognize the existence of the problem. Our own estimate is that three out of every four of our patients suffer from some form of sensitivity. These people, of course, have become aware that they have a problem and alarmed enough to seek help. It is likely that an equal percentage of those who chronically feel under par or who suffer an occasional symptom, but who are not concerned enough to visit a doctor's office, are similarly burdened by sensitivities.

What Is Brain Sensitivity?

Brain sensitivity has been implicated in a whole series of major and minor problems. Its symptoms can range from mild and barely noticeable irritations to acute forms of psychosis. It has been known to cause small discomforts (occasional listlessness, mild insomnia), mild reactions (minor headaches, irritability, restlessness), more severe symptoms (anxiety, depression, outbursts of violence, migraines, defects in memory), and even problems that are clearly psychotic (hallucinations, catatonia). Its symptoms can be either emotional or physical, and they can involve practically any part of the brain.

Brain sensitivity is often caused by foods, but can stem from inhalants and chemicals as well. The foods most commonly suspect are those most frequently eaten—namely, milk, wheat and corn and their products.

How does brain sensitivity fit into our modern concept of disease? At one time, people believed that most illnesses arose from inside the body as spirits and "bad vapors," and that only some of the more obvious exceptions—such as bubonic plague and syphilis—came from external sources. But within the past one hundred years, our understanding of illness and disease has changed completely. After Louis Pasteur's research into disease-causing bacteria, people began to realize that many illnesses were caused not by some internal problem but by an invasion from without. With the discovery of allergies some thirty years later, we began to understand that problems could also be caused by things in our environment that were larger than germs, things that were visible and familiar to everyone. The vulnerability of some people to various foods, from strawberries to shellfish, also demonstrated that anyone can be allergic or sensitive to elements in our environment that otherwise seem completely harmless.

The concept of brain sensitivity becomes clearer if we examine these better-known sensitivities. It is common knowledge, for example, that people who are sensitive or allergic to certain foods break out in hives or rashes when they eat them. Because the rashes or hives affect the skin, such reactions are considered to be skin sensitivities or skin allergies. Another common example, hay fever, occurs when inhaled pollen affects the nasal passages. Some people with asthma may suffer an attack when they eat a food or inhale a chemical to which they are sensitive. In each of these situations the reaction to the toxic substance is restricted to a single part of the body. Thus it is generally true that an allergic reaction causing asthma does not affect the skin or the sinuses; an attack of hay fever usually leaves the lungs and skin alone; and strawberries may cause an individual to break out in hives, but there is no involvement of the sinuses or lungs.

It is clear, then, that the body can respond selectively (that is, with only one organ or system) to allergenic or sensitizing substances, and that any given substance tends repeatedly to affect the same part of the body.

Clinical experience has shown that it is not just the skin, the lungs, or the sinuses that may become involved; any part of the body—including the brain—may be affected. We have seen cases of sensitivity in which the knees and knuckles have exhibited symptoms mimicking arthritic conditions; in which the kidneys were affected, causing sudden and dramatic weight gain as a result of fluid accumulation; and in which the vocal cords were attacked, resulting in hoarseness.

Our primary concern in this book, however, is with the brain and with problems that result from the brain's having become sensitive to one or more foods or chemicals. When such a sensitivity occurs, the condition is called a brain sensitivity or a cerebral allergy.

Technically, the term cerebral allergy is somewhat of a misnomer, because the sensitivities we are discussing do not necessarily fit the strictest medical (immunological) definition of allergy, although from a clinical point of view they behave much like classical allergies. One factor that separates a brain sensitivity from some of the more recognized allergies is that it generally has a second component: an addiction to the very substance that is causing the sensitivity.

Traditionally, a person who has an allergy to strawberries which causes him to break out in hives, doesn't develop a physical need for the fruit. However, when the brain is involved, people who are affected develop an actual craving for the food to which they are sensitive. They may even experience symptoms of withdrawal whenever they do not ingest it. And the symptoms of withdrawal can be worse than the symptoms caused by the intake of the addicting agent itself.

Let's use alcohol as an illustration. Those who are capable of drinking an alcoholic beverage once in a while without any adverse effects are not addicted and are probably not sensitive to alcohol. However, for alcoholics, chronic drinking can bring on a variety of symptoms. One reason that alcoholics drink—and keep on drinking—is to stave off those awful shakes, sweats, nightmares and hallucinations that result from withdrawal.

Similarly, brain sensitivity is a cross between an allergy and an addiction. Its symptoms can be brought on by eating a certain food (allergy component); yet, even worse symptoms can appear when that food is not eaten (withdrawal component). As with alcohol, the withdrawal symptoms can often be alleviated by eating the food again (addictive component). That is why so many people are surprised to learn that they are sensitive to such things as coffee, sugar or milk. They insist that the results of the testing must be wrong, because the substance in question happens to be the very one they use to ease the worst symptoms whenever they occur!

This, then, is the vicious cycle of sensitivity: You can become sensitive to certain foods; periods of withdrawal tell you that those foods can lessen your symptoms and make you feel better; the foods become favorites and are incorporated into your diet on a regular basis; and, after a while, meals seem incomplete without the bread, cola, coffee or green pepper that ends the headache, sleeplessness or anxiety.

As you eat foods to which you are unknowingly sensitive (called *hidden* or *masked* food sensitivities), subtle damage is taking place in your body. Even as the foods make you feel better by relieving withdrawal symptoms, the damage is intensifying. Hidden or masked food sensitivities can go unnoticed for a long time, as they did in the case of Mr. C.

A BEDTIME STORY

Mr. C was a hard-working executive. Because there were rarely enough hours in the day for him, he usually brought his work home—work that primarily involved reading he had to do to stay abreast of new developments in his field. As a general rule he would spend the early part of the evening with his family, then begin reading somewhere between 10 and 11 P.M. Invariably he found himself unable to concentrate for more than an hour before he began to feel sleepy. This pattern continued for several years, yet never did it occur to Mr. C that his inability to stay awake at these times was in any way abnormal. He simply assumed that, after getting up early and putting in a full day's work, he would naturally become sleepy when he tried to read at night.

Knowing nothing about brain sensitivity, Mr. C decided for reasons of his own to try a few days of fasting. During this period he continued his regular work routine. He felt drained and tired on the second day of his fast, but became invigorated on the third day. On the evening of the third day he sat down to read at 11 P.M., fully expecting to read no more than forty-five minutes or so before his eyes would begin to close. At the end of an hour he was still going strong. Without a trace of sleepiness, he read for three hours and finally went to bed, not because of his usual exhaustion but because it was 2 A.M. This newfound energy remained with him throughout the fast and for a few days thereafter.

Then he noticed, totally on his own, that when he ate foods loaded with sugar, his old pattern of sleepiness would return; when he avoided those foods, he could read for considerably longer periods.

Mr. C was aware that he relied on sweets for quick bursts of energy when he felt tired during the day, but he had not made the connection between his eating habits and his falling asleep while reading. The fast he undertook actually unmasked a hidden sensitivity to sugar. Shortly thereafter, he met us and told us of his spontaneous diagnosis of a brain sensitivity.

Many people have problems similar to Mr. C's. Often a tired feeling comes after lunch. Since the sensation doesn't surface until an hour or more after eating, they don't connect it with what they have eaten; they simply assume that they need a coffee break —perhaps with a candy bar—and they go on to supply themselves with precisely the food to which they are sensitive to avoid symptoms of withdrawal.

The Controversy

If brain sensitivity is as potent and widespread a condition as we have indicated, why has the medical community been so reluctant to recognize it? Following are some of the obstacles that have contributed to this reluctance.

1. MEDICAL LAG TIME

The medical community has a well-known, well-deserved reputation for taking a conservative stand on new or different forms of diagnosis, treatment and cure. The reason for this caution is clear: It would prefer that methods which sound superficially appealing, but which are actually useless, remain outside of medical practice. This attitude has certainly kept some of the wilder medical extravagances out of widespread use, but it has also resulted in what is now seen as a "medical lag time" for sound but revolutionary ideas. From William Harvey, who suffered disgrace in the seventeenth century for his "absurd" notion that the heart pumped blood around the body through blood vessels, to Louis Pasteur, who was strongly criticized for suggesting that invisible microbes could be responsible for disease, the medical establishment has generally been unwilling to accept ideas that seemed at odds with its own beliefs.

In more recent years, medical orthodoxy leveled a barrage of criticism at Rachel Carson for her book *Silent Spring*, which pointed out the dangers of DDT and other pesticides. Since then DDT has been banned, and Ms. Carson's ideas have received widespread acceptance.

The record of the medical community on issues such as these makes it clear that it has a hard time learning from its mistakes. Medical lag time is as much a factor today as it ever was.

2. CLINICAL IMMUNOLOGY VERSUS CLINICAL ECOLOGY

At the turn of the century, when allergies were first being investigated, researchers focused mainly on the relationship between certain environmental factors (like pollen) and their effects on people. The diseases that were related to allergy were those that we usually think of as allergic in nature, namely, hay fever, asthma and eczema. As the years went by, research in allergy was concentrated on these diseases and on the changes that took place in the body when allergic reactions developed. These reactions were found to involve the body's immune mechanism (for example, the production of antibodies in response to allergens). The allergists who were strongly influenced by this approach became known as clinical immunologists.

About the same time clinical immunology was getting started, another group of allergists began to expand the realm of allergy by observing that food reactions could cause a wide variety of symptoms involving the brain and other organ systems. This second group, known as clinical ecologists, were not so much concerned with the internal changes that accompanied an allergic reaction as they were with relationships between environmental (or ecological) factors—such as food—and the allergic response. But the emphasis on the body's internal response has continued to dominate the field of allergy; and since the internal mechanisms of brain sensitivity for the most part have not yet been demonstrated, most clinical immunologists tend to ignore their role in the formation of symptoms. Instead, they generally regard what we believe to be brain sensitivity reactions as psychological in origin.

3. FIXED FOOD SENSITIVITIES VERSUS CYCLIC FOOD SENSITIVITIES

All physicians—clinical immunologists and clinical ecologists included—concur that food allergies do exist. They all agree, for example, that there are people who develop hives every time they eat strawberries or shellfish. Clinical ecologists, however, believe that these fixed food allergies comprise perhaps only five percent of all food allergies and that the vast majority of sensitivities are not fixed but cyclic food allergies.

Someone who is suffering from a cyclic allergy to a particular food may react differently at different times; sometimes he may not react at all. Whether a reaction surfaces or not is dependent on a number of factors, including the amount of stress the individual is subjected to when he is exposed. This inconsistent pattern makes it difficult for scientists and physicians to accept the concept of cyclic allergies. That they do exist, however, is clearly illustrated by the following case of Gladys.

A DIZZY DAME

Gladys was an aspiring actress who came to see us because of periodic attacks of vertigo—sudden, recurring bouts of dizziness from which she had been suffering for two and a half years. During these attacks the room seemed to spin, and she was unable to walk or stand; even when sitting she had to hold on to something to keep from falling off the chair. Often she heard a ringing noise. These episodes lasted from a few minutes to an hour or so and were completely unpredictable.

Gladys consulted a neurologist and an ear, nose and throat specialist. Neither found anything wrong with her, and both recommended that she get psychiatric help.

A careful evaluation of her history made us suspect a brain sensitivity. Kinesiologic testing (see Chapter Five) revealed a sensitivity to chocolate. When we advised her to abstain from it, she protested. First of all, she maintained, she loved chocolate; and second, she knew that chocolate was definitely not the cause of her vertigo because she could recall many instances of having eaten it without any dizziness. As a matter of fact, although the attacks did generally occur three or four times a week, she ate chocolate just about every day. Convinced that logic was on her side, she refused to go along with our advice; but she did agree to watch her eating habits to see if she could discern any relationship between her diet and her attacks of vertigo.

We didn't see Gladys for another four months, at which time she returned and announced that she had not had an attack of vertigo for three months. She excitedly told us how she had made the discovery that we were right about the chocolate.

After her visit to our office, she had kept a log of what and when she ate, as well as a record of each vertigo attack. After two weeks the record confirmed her insistence that she often ate chocolate without any noticeable ill effects. On the other hand, each attack of vertigo was preceded by eating chocolate one to two hours beforehand. Therefore, chocolate seemed to relate to her dizzy spells, though inconsistently.

She puzzled over this while munching on a candy bar. That day passed without an attack. The next day she had an audition and had her usual pre-audition jitters. On the way to the theater she ate some chocolate to calm herself. She felt she did well at the audition, but on the way home she had a vertigo attack. (It was about two hours since she had eaten the chocolate.) After this attack it occurred to her that her nervousness may have contributed to it. Gladys then altered her record-keeping to note what and when she ate on one side of a page and her activities on the other side. Vertigo attacks were indicated by red stars. Within a week the situation became clear. Neither chocolate nor tension alone resulted in vertigo, but the combination of the two invariably did. Concluding that it was easier to give up chocolate than to avoid stress, Gladys managed to prevent any further bouts of vertigo.

4. BRAIN SENSITIVITY AS AN ACCOMPLISHED MIMIC

Mimics are not at all new to medicine. One of the best-known is syphilis, which in its prime (before the discovery of antibiotics) was often referred to as "the great imitator." When syphilis was running rampant, a patient could go to the doctor's office complaining of everything from body sores to pains in his liver, from arthritis to hallucinations. Yet all these symptoms could, and often did, have syphilis as a common cause.

Because brain sensitivities can affect different portions of the brain, they mimic many psychiatric, neurological and physical syndromes. In fact, brain sensitivity often imitates what are generally considered to be classical psychiatric problems so well that, clinically, the two look exactly the same; anxiety is anxiety, whether it is caused by a sensitivity or by an Oedipal complex. The same holds true for depression, irritability, hallucinations and bouts of violence. And the better the mimic, the more difficult it is to recognize. (For an extensive list of possible symptoms, see Appendix 1.)

It Started in Brooklyn

The idea of brain sensitivity must seem a far cry from the teachings of traditional psychiatry. So how did two physicians from Brooklyn with orthodox psychiatric training and background get involved with something like food sensitivities?

Although it now seems only natural to us that the food we eat and other environmental factors can have a profound influence on our mental state, we were not always aware of this connection. These ideas were, in fact, far from our minds when we first met during our psychiatric residency training at Kings County Hospital in Brooklyn, New York.

The residency program at Kings County emphasized the Freudian analytic approach to psychiatry. In addition, we both undertook more advanced psychoanalytic studies. Our goal was to become classical psychoanalysts, and we might well have gone that route had it not been for Vietnam and the United States Government's feeling that we could both better serve our country in Mississippi.

Through some quirk of fate, both of us ended up in the air force, stationed at the same base, and jointly assigned to direct a large psychiatric outpatient clinic. It was here that a totally different phase of our psychiatric education began.

Long-term psychoanalytic treatment, which up until then had been the approach we favored, was not well suited to the military need for rapid resolution of problems. As a result, we began to search for new, presumably more effective therapeutic techniques by attending workshops in different parts of the country. Through this process we found that there were, in fact, many potent and valuable therapeutic techniques available, and we began to learn about treatment methods such as behavioral therapy, transactional analysis, gestalt therapy and bioenergetic analysis.

The last two of these therapeutic techniques taught us that in psychiatry it is sometimes as important to work with the body as it is with the mind. It seemed a novel idea to us that one's personality could be reflected as much by the structure of one's body as it could by one's mind. But if we had looked closely at our profession's past, it would not have seemed strange at all.

Psychoanalysis had its origin in Freud's attempts to understand physical disturbances in the body. His first psychoanalytic cases, in fact, dealt with "hysterical" bodily symptoms (such as paralysis) that occurred even though there was no neurological disease present. As it continued its development, psychiatry could never dissociate itself from these physical manifestations of emotional conflict; nevertheless, the predominant psychiatric attitude has always been to consider the psychic causes of these conflicts. Some of the newer therapies we studied accepted this approach, but they added the possibility that these conflicts had their physical causes as well. The newer therapies operated on the premise that whatever affects us is ultimately reflected both in the mind and in the body. This novel way of thinking expanded our own arsenal of treatments and opened our minds to the potential value of unconventional approaches to therapy.

As we look back, it is interesting that although we came to appreciate the role of the body in the development of emotional symptoms, we gave little clinical thought to the food, air and water the body consumed. A problem with legs finally opened our eyes.

The legs belonged to a woman who had a bad case of phlebitis (an inflammation of the veins). She was the daughter of one of our secretaries, and she asked our advice because she was not responding well to traditional medical treatment. Unfortunately we knew of no treatment other than the traditional, and we were unable to help her. We were very surprised a few weeks later when the secretary gleefully announced that her daughter's phlebitis had disappeared. We were even more surprised when she told us what her daughter had done to accomplish this. Someone had told her that vitamin E was an effective treatment for phlebitis; she had taken vitamin E, and the problem had cleared up.

We had heard of other cases in which cures, both miraculous and mundane, were attributed to vitamins, but our ignorance and prejudices had kept us from researching them. This case was not particularly unusual in the annals of nutritional therapy, but it was the first in our own experience. It launched what was to become an intense interest in the fields of nutrition and ecology as they relate to illness and health.

It was later, at one of the many medical conferences and workshops on nutritional therapy we attended, that we first heard of brain sensitivity. Brain sensitivity wasn't a major topic of discussion then; it was only casually mentioned by a psychiatrist in the audience who stood up to ask a question of a speaker. It didn't strike us as particularly momentous, and we gave it little thought.

In fact, the idea that one's brain could become sensitive to foods or chemicals, and that such a sensitivity could be responsible for a whole host of emotional symptoms, remained somewhere in the backs of our minds—until we encountered the milkman.

In this book we shall discuss brain sensitivity and the various methods of diagnosing it—at home and in the laboratory. We shall also look into how it can be treated, and how rational management of our diets can literally change our lives. But first let's examine in more depth the evidence for brain sensitivity.

TWO:
Crackpot Theory
or Established Fact?

The concept of brain sensitivity may sound radical, an idea drawn from the revelations of the fairly recent movement for health through nutrition. But it is actually derived from observations and practices that are as old as medicine itself.

One of the first physicians to recognize the connection between what we eat and how we feel was Hippocrates. Over two thousand years ago, Hippocrates observed and described how cheese upset some people and not others. In his writings he also demanded that physicians understand not only the inner workings of the human body, but the relationship of man to his environment, to the things he eats and drinks, and to his daily activities. In the lovely, rounded style of ancient Greece, he recognized the connection between disease and incorrect diet:

> Such persons, provided they take dinner when it is not their wont, immediately become heavy and inactive, both in body and in mind, and are weighed down with yawning, slumbering and thirst; and if they take supper in addition, they are seized with flatulence, yormina and diarrhea, and to many this has been the commencement of a serious disease, when they have merely taken twice a day the same food which they have been in the custom of taking once.

Hippocrates was certainly not the last physician before modern times to study the effects of food upon health. But until the nineteenth century, food took a back seat as a causative factor in illness (unless, of course, it was poisoned or spoiled). Most studies of starvation and of diseases like scurvy and beriberi concerned themselves with the lack of certain foods and important nutrients and with our dependence on food for our health and well-being. It was only in the latter part of the last century that researchers began to discover connections among food, allergies and behavioral abnormalities.

Once those connections did surface, other observations followed. Publications noted the links between grass pollen and listlessness, food allergies and behavioral disturbances, and allergy and tension. In 1889 Dr. Francis Hare observed that migraines could be relieved when patients were placed on diets which "largely excluded fats, carbohydrates and saccharine alcoholic drinks. . . ." In 1908 Dr. Schofield of England immunized a thirteen-year-old boy who suffered from swelling and asthma as a result of an allergy to eggs. And in 1924 Seale Harris, writing in the *Journal of the American Medical Association,* clearly showed the relationship between certain foods (like sugar) and behavioral abnormalities in his classic paper describing functional hypoglycemia.

Research into food and its connection with allergy continued to result in new discoveries. In 1931 Albert Rowe published the first major work on the subject: *Food Allergy (Its Manifestations, Diagnosis and Treatment).* In it Rowe provided evidence that food allergies were primary causes of bronchial asthma, obstructive emphysema, gastric and abdominal allergies, ulcerative colitis, nasal allergy, eczema, headaches, fatigue, and urogenital and musculoskeletal reactions.

About the time Rowe published his findings, another doctor, Herbert Rinkel, was himself suffering greatly from continual headaches, severe nasal congestion and fatigue. His condition had begun several years before and had worsened as he grew older. Determined to improve his health, Rinkel read some of Rowe's material and wondered whether a food allergy could be contributing to his condition. Suspecting eggs, which he ate daily, he ate six at one time, fully expecting his symptoms to worsen; but much to his chagrin, he actually felt better. Rinkel therefore concluded that he was not allergic to eggs.

Four years later, as his symptoms grew worse, Rinkel decided to try eliminating eggs from his diet. After several days he began to feel better. About a week later, while eating cake that his wife had baked, he suddenly collapsed. Suspecting that he had reacted to something in the cake, Rinkel checked the ingredients and learned that they included eggs. As a result of his experience, Rinkel developed the concept of masked or hidden food allergies, which could be discovered if the food in question was eaten after a period of abstinence.

During World War II, Dr. Theron Randolph, who currently practices medicine in Chicago, was skin-testing soldiers for allergies to various substances. During the testing, Randolph noticed that many of the soldiers would fall asleep or would become irritable while waiting for the tests to be completed. These signs showed up both in soldiers with positive skin reactions and in those without them. Other physicians had performed similar tests and had noticed the same phenomena, but to them it seemed normal that a soldier would react in this way under such conditions.

Randolph, however, focused on these odd reactions. He retested some of the soldiers and found that the irritation or sleepiness did not surface just because the men were involved in testing, but only when they were exposed to specific substances. Thus the idea that allergenic substances could affect behavior rather than simply cause such physical reactions as rashes and asthma was reinforced.

Today, after thirty more years of clinical research into the subject of brain sensitivities, we find evidence of their existence in three forms: in double-blind studies, the kinds of testing most often relied on by modern researchers; in the clinical experience of physicians who have been working with the concept of brain sensitivity for years; and in the personal experiences of lay people, both patients and other individuals, who have spontaneously recognized that they feel depressed after drinking milk or sleepy after eating green peppers.

Crackpot theory or established fact? Let's examine the evidence that has been building over the years in favor of the existence of brain sensitivity.

Double-Blind Studies

What exactly are double-blind studies? Let's look at a specific example. Suppose a pharmaceutical company wants to test the effectiveness of a drug that may be used to treat schizophrenia, a form of mental illness. A number of schizophrenics (who have been carefully chosen for the study and who have given their informed consent) are divided into two groups, matched as closely as possible for age, sex, socioeconomic variables, nature and severity of symptoms, and other relevant factors. The researchers observe various kinds of behavioral symptoms of anxiety and depression, level of activity, social avoidance and hallucinations during the experiment to determine whether the schizophrenics improve under the influence of the new drug.

One of the two groups is given the drug to be tested—Drug X. The other is given a capsule which looks exactly the same, but which contains an inert substance and is called a placebo. Neither the patients nor the doctors administering the drugs know who is receiving what. (A single-blind study is one in which it is only the patients who don't know who is getting the drug and who isn't.) Then, for a specified period of time, Drug X and the placebo are administered, and the patients' reactions are observed and recorded.

Double-blind studies are conducted mainly because researchers have found that the high expectations of either the patient or the doctor can influence the effectiveness of almost any drug or program. This so-called placebo effect has been demonstrated many times. In one example, teachers were told that certain children in their classes were highly gifted, as reflected in their IQ tests. The children were actually chosen on a random basis without regard to actual test scores. By the end of the school year the performances of the selected children were far above those expected for children not influenced by teacher expectations.

Over the past thirty years the double-blind study has become an integral part of medical research, so much so that some doctors reject any new idea that is not supported by these studies. Recently, however, the efficacy of the double-blind study itself has been questioned.

Among the criticisms leveled at this type of study are: (1) The very conditions which make studies double blind are so different from conditions under which treatment is usually administered that the results noted in the former may actually be different from the results obtained in a more typical patient-doctor setting. For example, in a clinical setting, both the physician and the patient work toward the mutual goal of helping the patient—a situation which inspires rapport and mutual trust. In the double-blind situation, the primary goal is to experiment, to learn whether a treatment is effective, and not necessarily to help the patient. This setting tends to inspire distrust and confusion. (2) Although the double-blind study may be suitable for testing an individual drug, it is not suitable for testing an entire complicated treatment approach which has many variables capable of influencing one another. (3) The physician cannot tailor the dosage of the drug to his patient. (4) Only certain types of patients will voluntarily participate in such a study; thus, a bias is introduced into the experiment.

The objections to double-blind studies make it clear that they are not the panaceas some researchers would have us believe. Nevertheless, they have been used to shed light on the relationships among food, brain sensitivity, and certain disorders, as seen in the following three double-blind studies.

1. THE LAND OF MILK AND WHEAT

The first study was performed at a Veterans Administration Hospital in Pennsylvania by Dohan and Grassberger, and the results were published in a series of articles in well-respected psychiatric journals. The subjects were 150 male veterans who had been diagnosed as schizophrenic and whose symptoms were so severe that they had been confined to a locked ward. For this study the clinicians and patients were told that the patients would be divided into two random groups. The experimental group received a diet devoid of wheat gluten and dairy products, whereas the control group was given the regular hospital diet, which was high in gluten and milk products. Unbeknownst to either the patients or the clinicians, there was a secret third group. This group constituted a portion of the experimental group who were supposed to be getting a diet free of gluten and milk products, but wheat gluten was secretly added to their muffins. Since neither the patients nor the clinicians were aware of the gluten in the muffins, this group constituted a double-blind control group.

The patients continued their diets only while they were on the locked wards. When they had shown sufficient improvement, they were reassigned to open wards and given regular diets.

The results of the study were clear. Patients receiving the gluten- and milk-free diets were discharged from the locked ward in about half the time it took for the other two groups to be discharged. Furthermore, the therapeutic effect of the diet appeared to last for as long as ninety days after it was discontinued, as was evidenced by earlier discharge from the hospital.

2. THE ELECTRIC KOOL-AID TEST

Another double-blind study was carried out at the Bronx Psychiatric Center by Singh and Kay.

Fourteen severely ill schizophrenic patients were evaluated carefully by trained observers for fourteen weeks. During this time their hospital diet was supposed to be free from all gluten and dairy products. Each patient received a daily Kool-Aid drink containing soy powder (which contains no gluten) during both the first six weeks and the last four weeks of the study. But without the knowledge of either patients or staff, wheat gluten flour was substituted for the soy flour during weeks seven through ten.

An analysis of the results clearly showed that the patients

improved when their diet was free of milk and gluten, but that they stopped improving or became worse when the gluten flour was secretly added. When the gluten was again removed, their improvement continued.

This study is extremely significant, because the investigators were able to show a clear relationship between gluten ingestion and schizophrenic deterioration. (One wonders if the results would have been even more dramatic if the investigators had eliminated the artificial coloring, flavoring and sugar found in both the Kool-Aid and the regular hospital diet.)

3. OKAY, FORGET THE LOBOTOMY

An interesting and dramatic double-blind study of a single case is described by Dr. Richard Mackarness, an ecologically oriented psychiatrist from England, in his book *Eating Dangerously.*

The patient, 28-year-old Joanna D., had been admitted to Park Prewitt Psychiatric Hospital twelve times over a five-year period. Following the birth of her third child in 1967 she became irritable, depressed, unable to feed her baby, and occasionally violent toward her two older children. For this condition she was given electroshock therapy at another hospital. Subsequently, she was hospitalized at Park Prewitt, frequently involuntarily, because she was a danger both to herself and to her children. "In her most disturbed phases she would slash her forearms with any available sharp object, not with definite suicidal intent but as a way of relieving, if only temporarily, the unbearable tension and irritability mounting inside her. These wounds usually needed stitching and left deep scars. . . ." After every available treatment—including psychotherapy, various drugs, and electroshock therapy—proved unsuccessful, the doctors agreed that Joanna D. needed a frontal lobotomy.

Dr. Mackarness, who had been exposed to the work of Dr. Theron Randolph and other clinical ecologists, recommended that the patient be tested for brain sensitivity before the lobotomy. With little to lose, the skeptical doctors reluctantly agreed to Dr. Mackarness's plan.

Joanna fasted on spring water for several days. Within two or three days she had begun to show improvement, and by the end of five days she was symptom-free. She was then given test helpings of single foods over the next week or two. Severe reactions occurred with seven foods: bacon, eggs, oatmeal, veal, tongue, instant coffee and chocolate.

To rule out the possibility that her improvement was due to the power of suggestion, ten foods were tested in a double-blind fashion. Over a ten-day period the dietitian made up liquid solutions of five of the foods to which Joanna had reacted and five foods to which she had not. The foods were administered through a tube inserted into Joanna's stomach through her nose, and were delivered in syringes which were covered to conceal their contents. Thus, neither the investigator nor the patient knew what she was receiving. Joanna reacted severely to five of the foods. When the code was finally broken, it turned out that she had reacted only to the foods that previous testing had implicated and not to those believed harmless. Thereafter, Joanna continued to remain free of symptoms without medication as long as she avoided the offending foods.

Clinical Experience

Clinical experience with brain sensitivity has been accumulating for three decades. There are now scores of physicians in this country who have encountered brain sensitivities, recognized them for what they are, and treated them successfully.

Clinical evidence in itself does not satisfy the passion of modern science and medicine for controlled, reproducible experiments. Because it is colored by such variables as the placebo effect of the doctor-patient relationship, the lack of adequate control over the patient's environment, and the desire of some physicians to discover new and different approaches to medical problems (a situation that might cause them to see things where they do not exist), modern medicine accepts clinical reports mainly as preliminary findings on a particular problem, and then sits back to await the results of "more conclusive" studies, such as double-blind experiments. Nevertheless, clinical experience does have value and should not be summarily dismissed.

Let's look at a few of the more clear-cut cases we have seen over the years. Most of our cases of brain sensitivity have been diagnosed only after they had resisted the usual methods of diagnosis and treatment offered by other clinicians; most have been helped through some relatively simple yet direct steps that many orthodox medical practitioners would consider to be benign but useless.

JACK BE NIMBLE, JACK BE QUICK . . .

Sister Jacqueline was a member of a religious order. She had a reputation for being one of the most dedicated and hard-working members of her community. Then, rather suddenly, she became ill. The only real symptoms of her illness were a loss of energy and feelings of fatigue and listlessness. Sister Jacqueline felt so weak that she spent a good part of her day dragging herself through her chores. This lack of energy was completely out of character. When her superiors learned of it, they became alarmed and sought medical help.

Over the next six years Sister Jacqueline was examined by a dozen physicians. She underwent batteries of tests and scores of specialized examinations. Nothing the doctors did, however, uncovered any underlying abnormality. Finally, one of the physicians concluded that her problem might be emotional rather than physical and suggested that she seek psychiatric help.

By the time Sister Jacqueline came to see us, her medical chart was as thick as a New York City telephone directory, yet nothing in it gave us a clue as to what was wrong with her. As we listened to her history, however, it struck us that her complaints were clearly consistent with a diagnosis of brain sensitivity. We had learned by then that the brain could become sensitive not only to foods but to chemicals in the environment as well. Since Sister Jacqueline was regularly exposed to a number of chemicals (including various solutions used to clean her living quarters), we knew that it would be important to test her for sensitivity to them.

As we suspected, the tests revealed sensitivities to both foods and chemicals. With great confidence we announced that we had found the physical problem causing the symptoms; if Sister Jacqueline avoided the things to which she was sensitive, we were sure her symptoms would disappear—or at least diminish—in a relatively short time.

Having spent years disciplining herself, Sister Jacqueline assured us that she would do everything she could to avoid the foods and chemicals that we had labeled as sensitizing; and for the next several weeks she followed our program faithfully.

She did not, however, improve one bit. Her symptoms continued unabated, the placebo effect notwithstanding. It seemed as if we would finally have to abandon the idea that Sister Jacqueline's problem had a physical cause.

But something about the case told us not to give up on the physical possibilities so quickly, and we again asked Sister Jacqueline and her Mother Superior to describe in detail Sister Jacqueline's activities from morning to night. Nothing new emerged from the discussion. Commenting that they would consider beginning psychotherapy, the two nuns thanked us and headed for the door. As they were leaving the office, the Mother Superior turned to Sister Jacqueline and said something about going back, praying for guidance, and lighting an extra candle.

Up to that point nothing had been mentioned about candles, and we hurriedly called them back. It was only then that they explained that it was their custom before going to sleep to light a candle at their bedsides and to leave it burning all night long.

We sent for a candle, lit it, and had Sister Jacqueline inhale the hydrocarbon fumes. Within moments she was feeling a marked intensification of the symptoms with which she had been struggling for six years.

Early in our consultation Sister Jacqueline had mentioned that her symptoms were always worse in the morning, then eased as the day progressed. Depression due to psychological factors often follows a similar pattern: an individual may wake up feeling that he doesn't have the strength to get out of bed and face another day. When he finally does get up, his depression eases, and it continues to improve as the day goes on.

Although Sister Jacqueline's symptoms could have been explained away as part of such a depression, it turned out that in fact her brain had become sensitive to the fumes she was inhaling during the night. By morning she was literally drugged and unable to function. As the day went on she gained strength, but at night she again breathed in the sensitizing chemicals produced by the burning candle. That is how her symptoms had been perpetuated from day to day for six years. When candles were removed from her living and working areas, she became stronger by the day. Within ten days she was completely symptom-free. She has since returned to her previous level of dedicated hard work and has remained free of her symptoms for the past two years.

Sister Jacqueline's case has much to teach us, not the least of which is the importance of paying attention to minute details when searching for sensitizing agents. Just as Sister Jacqueline's symptoms were related to the inhalation of candle fumes, symptoms could result from other sources of hydrocarbons such as the new vinyl tiles in your bathroom, the cleaning agents used to wash your floors, or your auto exhaust, particularly if your garage is under your bedroom. In treating brain sensitivities, as in treating skin allergies, good detective work is often an essential ingredient.

WHAT HAPPENED TO SUNDAY?

One of our most ironic case histories began with the writing of this book. Our collaborator, Richard Hutton, had been working with us for several weeks, gathering material and joining in our discussions. One day, out of the blue, he mentioned that the symptoms we were describing seemed to apply to him as well; he had felt chronically listless and tired for several years. His symptoms were not very strong; they only nudged the edge of his awareness. Nevertheless, he had discussed them with a physician friend and had received the typical reply: "You're probably overworked and feeling the pressure."

We decided to test Richard cytotoxically (see Chapter Six) to see what we could find. Sure enough, his tests showed that he was sensitive to wheat and green peppers. Kinesiologic tests (see Chapter Five) confirmed those findings.

Curious, Richard decided to go along with our recommendation to eliminate wheat and green peppers from his diet. After following this routine for a month, he found that his listlessness did indeed disappear. Then, one Saturday, someone invited him out to an Italian restaurant for dinner.

If there is one food Richard is passionate about, it is fettucine Alfredo. That night, with the prospect of velvety noodles in a cheese and butter sauce staring him in the face, he persuaded himself that the tests were wrong. He ordered the fettucine and cleaned his plate.

He went home that night feeling fine. After what seemed like a decent night's sleep, he was awakened by a phone call. It was a friend, asking him why he had skipped their breakfast appointment.

"What appointment?" asked Richard, obviously confused. "We were supposed to meet on Monday."

His friend was not amused. It took her five minutes to convince him that he had slept right through Sunday, and that it was, indeed, Monday morning.

Sister Jacqueline and Richard represent examples of brain sensitivities occurring in adults. But children are just as susceptible to brain sensitivities. We have worked with quite a few children whose emotional problems, hyperactive behavior, and learning disabilities were directly related to sensitivities. Where these disorders do result from a brain sensitivity, removing the offending agents from a child's environment results in the same kind of improvement in the child as in adults.

THE CANDY MAN CAN

By the time John was nine years old, he had been evaluated by school and private psychiatrists and psychologists. He was described by his teachers as above average in ability but decidedly hyperactive. He tended to be aggressive and was quick to strike out in response to frustrating situations. He was unable to sit in his chair in class or to concentrate for any length of time; therefore, despite his ability, his school work was poor. As one of his psychological evaluators observed, "He was almost uncontrollably hyperactive. He handled test material without permission, and he became aggressive at times against objects in the room. Speech was noted to be immature."

Four years later John's mother came to see us in the hope that we might be able to help her son. She preferred not to have John take medication on a daily basis unless it was absolutely essential.

Laboratory testing revealed that John had a number of metabolic imbalances. To correct them, we recommended a nutritional program that eliminated "junk foods" such as those containing refined sugar, artificial flavoring, artificial coloring and preservatives. Of course John was not in favor of such a program, but his mother was determined to give it a try. Within a few weeks his mother noted a marked improvement in John's behavior and disposition. Although pleased, we were not surprised. Dr. Ben Feingold and others had demonstrated that many children are hyperactive as a result of a sensitivity to certain artificial additives, as well as to natural foods containing salicylates. (See Appendix 5.) Our own clinical experience had also borne this out.

John and his mother were surprised at the rapid change in John's behavior. John, however, missed many of his old foods and refused to believe that his getting better had anything to do with his diet. He particularly rebelled at giving up his favorite sweets. The turning point came when he managed, without his parents' knowledge, to eat a dozen candy bars over a two-week period. John's parents reported a "dreadful change in him. . . . He became completely hyperactive and in truth unbearable." After considerable detective work, the cause of this relapse was uncovered. John emerged from the experience with an awareness that certain foods could turn his whole world upside down. What neither we nor his parents could impress upon him, John learned from the Candy Man.

Personal Experiences

Many people come in contact with examples of brain sensitivity every day—in themselves, their relatives, their friends, or their co-workers. Think about it for a minute. Do you know someone who gets cranky or irritable within a few hours of eating, who seems to need coffee or candy or bread—or some other type of food—more than others do, and is seldom satisfied unless that food has been part of his or her meal? Or, do you know someone who reacts strangely to the smell of burning fuel—gasoline or kerosene—or to the odor of cleaning fluids or synthetic fabrics? Because the idea of brain sensitivity is relatively new, and because so few medical practitioners are on the lookout for it, few people actually realize what they are seeing. They may attribute the mild or severe reaction they observe to an idiosyncrasy and may never associate it with a specific response to a food or a chemical.

Some, however, have had a different experience with brain sensitivity. Although they have not known it by name, they have become aware that specific reactions in themselves are somehow related to foods or to chemicals, and they have found their own ways of compensating for these sensitivities.

One such person who came to us as a patient was a rabbi. For most of his adult life, Rabbi L. had spent eight to twelve hours a day immersed in books. He did, however, take regular breaks during which he exercised. His main complaints centered around mental sluggishness, unclear thinking, and a lack of energy. He had discovered that these symptoms were made worse by eating. It seemed to make little difference what he ate; almost all foods seemed to aggravate the condition. When he ate a full meal, he invariably became sleepy within an hour or two. He had sought medical advice, but when both his physical examination and routine laboratory tests were found to be normal, he was told that there was nothing physically wrong with him. After hearing this from several doctors, he gave up on traditional medicine and decided to try to help himself.

Rabbi L. found that certain nutritional supplements, such as brewer's yeast, helped a little; but the greatest relief came from not eating at all. As a result, he generally avoided eating anything during the day and had only one large meal in the late evening. This pattern enabled him to get through the day, but it was obviously far from an ideal solution.

A detailed history, coupled with medical testing, indicated to us that Rabbi L. had multiple brain sensitivities. By following a careful plan of treatment and by avoiding certain key foods, Rabbi L. was able later to eat meals during the day without ill effects.

Many people have noted on their own that they develop symptoms such as headaches, pain or numbness in parts of their bodies, or difficulty in moving their jaws when they eat in Chinese restaurants. This phenomenon, often called "Chinese restaurant syndrome," has a known cause: MSG. Monosodium glutamate is an additive used to accent the flavor of food. Many restaurants (and particularly Chinese restaurants) as well as home cooks use this product.

There are some people who develop symptoms from eating food containing MSG but, unless they know the additive is contained therein, will not link what they ate with how they feel later, since they don't always experience a reaction to the same food.

There are others who suffer from this reaction to MSG and who are aware of it. Some avoid eating in Chinese restaurants altogether; others eat Chinese cuisine only after requesting that MSG not be added to their food. One friend of ours is so fond of the food with the MSG added that he eats it despite the fact that his jaw is numb for a couple of hours afterwards. On several occasions we have been with him while he ate food laden with the additive. After two or three bites, he would begin to feel the numbness, but would just rub his jaw and continue eating. To him it was worth it.

We have now discussed what brain sensitivity is and how it might affect you. But simply knowing that it exists is not very useful. Fortunately, there are several ways to test for it. We shall discuss seven of these methods; three can be performed by you at home, and four must be performed in a doctor's office or a laboratory. Each test has its advantages and disadvantages (listed at the end of each discussion). Each can indicate whether or not you have brain sensitivities and, if so, to what you are sensitive.

Before we move on to testing, there are several important points to understand:

1. Sensitivities are often caused by foods, but can also be caused by chemicals and inhalants such as pollen and house dust. As a result, methods like fasting and deliberate food testing are effective for uncovering some of the possible sensitizing agents, but not all. (The uses to which each method can be put are described in each chapter.)

2. While the theory behind brain sensitivity is relatively simple, the problem itself can be complex. Some foods are actually a blend of basic foods, and you may be sensitive to any one of the ingredients. Other sensitivities may show up only when you are exposed to several toxic items at the same time.

3. The best way to decide which test will be appropriate for you is to read about all of them; then read through Chapter Seven, which describes factors that may complicate the testing. You will then be in a better position to decide which test is best suited to your individual needs.

Some sensitivities are complex; others are straightforward and simple. Let's look now at the seven methods of testing that will help you uncover sensitivities you might have.

THREE:
Fasting and Deliberate Food Testing

Fasting and deliberate food testing is a two-step procedure for uncovering food sensitivities. It involves a period of fasting, followed by a period of reintroducing foods one at a time. The rationale behind it is simple: symptoms caused by sensitivity to a food surface when the food is a part of your diet, disappear when it is discontinued, and reappear in intensified form when it is eaten a few days later. This method was the first that we used for diagnosing food sensitivities; it remains the most accurate and most reliable, serving as a standard by which other methods can be measured.

Fasting

When a person stops eating a food to which he has become sensitive, the symptoms may not disappear immediately, since traces of the food can remain in the body for days. In addition, avoiding a food to which we are sensitive can cause the withdrawal symptoms we discussed earlier. Therefore, in this method of testing for sensitivities, food must be completely eliminated for a period of four to ten days. For most people, four days is long enough. By abstaining from all food, we can be sure that the offending foods are being avoided. It may seem simpler and more to the point to eliminate just one suspected food rather than all foods. Although this form of deliberate food testing can work and is recommended in some cases, it has drawbacks, which we shall discuss later. Fasting also cleanses the body, making it more sensitive to the foods that will be tested later. This increased sensitivity enables you to detect reactions that might otherwise go unnoticed.

Most people instinctively stop eating when they feel sick and continue to avoid food until they are feeling better. Animals also fast when they are ill. It is clear that we are all equipped with an alarm system that takes away our appetite when we are sick.

Fasting has a long history behind it; it is one of the oldest known treatments for illness. The relationship between sickness and abstention from food is still an important factor in the practice of medicine, especially in the Soviet Union, China, and various European countries. In the Soviet Union psychiatric patients are encouraged to fast for as long as three weeks on admission to certain hospitals.

Despite medical and historical support, people are still suspicious of regulated fasting. The roots of this attitude seem to be cultural and psychological; having habitually eaten our three meals a day, we have somehow learned to equate fasting with starvation, and thus fasting has become associated in our minds with danger.

The differences between starving and fasting are, however, well defined. Fasting is generally voluntary; it is limited in time and can be ended at will; it is carried out for a specific purpose; and it is often associated with healing. Starvation, on the other hand, is generally forced; it is continued for an indefinite period of time and cannot be ended at will; it is not undertaken for purposes of healing; and it is generally harmful.

Fasting, as epitomized by the famous Swedish fast marches of the past (in which thirty men would walk from Gothenburg to Stockholm, a distance of over 325 miles, in ten days without eating anything), generally does not damage the body; rather, it usually has a revitalizing effect. As Dr. Karl-Otto Aly, a participant in one of the Swedish fast marches, noted: "The march clearly showed that man can live for an extended period of time without food, even accomplish a hard physical effort while fasting. The generally expressed feeling among participants was that they felt stronger and had more vigor and vitality after the fast than before it."

There are many reasons why fasting is beneficial for most people. First, during a fast your body begins to subsist on its own substance after a few days. But it doesn't simply burn its tissues indiscriminately; instead, it begins by decomposing and consuming cells and tissues that are already diseased, damaged, aging or dead. Second, the body's organs of elimination—lungs, liver, kidneys and skin—can detoxify the body more efficiently during a fast, since they aren't dealing with such an influx of new toxic material. And third, the various body systems are able to rest and recuperate from the day-in, day-out process of digesting and assimilating new food.

Fasting and deliberate food testing have been used as a tool to diagnose brain sensitivity in hospital ecological units in the United States for years. The hospital setting removes potentially confusing environmental variables and is therefore a purer way of testing. But fasting is also effective and safe for home tests. However, any fast of four or more days should be undertaken only under the supervision of a medical professional.

WHO SHOULD NOT FAST?

Medical research indicates that fasting is not dangerous for the normal, well-nourished individual. However, people who are severely rundown or undernourished should not fast for prolonged periods of time without first building up the body's store of nutrients (through vitamin and mineral supplements, for example). In addition, there exist a few diseases in which fasting is contraindicated. These include advanced cases of tuberculosis, active malignancies, advanced diabetes, and extreme emaciation or wasting diseases. All of these conditions leave the body without the stamina necessary to successfully complete a diagnostic water fast.

Others who should not fast are pregnant women, women who

have just given birth (particularly if they are nursing), and children, who need constant nourishment for growth. The elderly often go through long fasts without any problems at all. Generally, it is a good idea for everyone to prepare for his fast by having a complete physical checkup beforehand.

Finally, people with severe and chronic psychiatric problems such as schizophrenia and hallucinations should not fast without continual medical supervision.

PREPARING FOR THE FAST

It is best to ease into a fast by cutting down on the amount of food you eat for two or three days. Then, by the time the actual fast has started, the body will be prepared and the change will come as less of a shock. Some people, stocking up for the big deprivation, eat huge feasts on the eve of their fasts. But this only means that it will take longer for the fast to become effective.

Beginning a fast may sound like a big deal, but it doesn't necessarily have to be. Many people arrange their fasts around the weekend, when they will have the time and the energy to concentrate on them. They may begin Thursday evening, skip Friday breakfast, and then simply extend their abstention through the single working day. The problems of toxicity (discussed below) and withdrawal probably won't strike—if they strike at all—until late Friday or early Saturday, so they can deal with the less pleasant parts of the fast on nonworking days. A housewife may also find it easier to plan a fast in this way, when her husband will be home to help take care of the children. Also, there is usually more time to undertake some mild exercise such as walking, or to take a nap when one seems necessary, and to study carefully the changes one's body is experiencing. Then, by Monday, the worst is usually over. The fast has only one more day to run before the testing begins. (Of course, the subsequent testing may also elicit symptoms that will interfere with the normal schedule.)

Since water is the only substance a person should ingest during a diagnostic fast, he should make sure he is not sensitive to it. Several years ago one of our patients drank water from her own well during a fast. After four days she complained of feeling extremely lethargic. When we examined her, we found that she had developed an irregular heartbeat. At that point we tested her for sensitivity to her well water and found that she was in fact sensitive to substances in it. While fasting, she was taking in concentrated amounts of the very thing that was harming her.

Generally, spring water should be used during the fast. As a rule, we prefer to test our patients for sensitivity to water by kinesiology (see Chapter Five) to make sure the water they are to drink during their fasts is not harmful to them. If they cannot drink spring water, distilled water can be substituted.

Distilled or spring water should be kept in glass jugs or jars, since chemicals from plastic jugs may leach into the water during the storage period.

During the fast, exposure to chemical substances should be avoided as much as possible; in particular, smokers must avoid all forms of tobacco throughout this period of deliberate food testing.

KEEPING A JOURNAL

It can be very difficult to keep track of everything that goes on in a fast—when you drink water, when you experience symptoms of withdrawal or detoxification, or even when you begin to feel good again. So it is helpful to keep a journal.

During the fast, it is important to note any distinct changes you feel in your physical, mental or emotional state. Some will be relevant; some will be incidental. But all should be noted, along with the times that they occur. For example, if you suffer from headaches every night before bed, and if by the third day of the fast those headaches are gone, that is a significant indication of brain sensitivity. Or, if you tend to wake up feeling listless and tired, and if the feeling continues during the fast, note that your state has remained constant. If you write down your observations, you can look back after the testing and see whether there were indeed signs of sensitivity, and whether reactions which seemed important during the fast have lost their significance.

During deliberate food testing, keep records of your meals—what you ate, when you ate it, and how you felt afterwards. A small change that occurs when you eat chicken, for example, could take on added significance the next time you bite into a drumstick and remember that you felt a similar reaction during your testing. A brief muscle cramp, a momentary headache, a fleeting feeling of anxiety might be forgotten if it is not recorded. If your journal is complete, there is less chance that changes will escape your notice.

Marking down the time of day when something is eaten is also important. Some people seem to react to particular foods only at certain meals; at other times they can eat the same things and not develop symptoms. We know that there are all kinds of biorhythmic patterns, highs and lows of hormonal production, temperature changes, and other physical changes that take place in the body during the day, as well as differences in the amount of external stress and strain to which the body is subjected. Any or all of these factors may influence the degree to which you are sensitive, and an accurate journal will help to clarify these relationships.

THE FAST

A fast has three phases. In the first, you should experience little reaction except, perhaps, hunger pangs. In the second phase, you enter a period of withdrawal and/or detoxification and may feel worse than you felt before you began the fast. And in the third phase, you begin to feel a sense of well-being, as both your chronic sensitivity reactions and your symptoms of withdrawal and detoxification have disappeared. Although these phases generally occur within a four-day period, their length may vary considerably from person to person. As a general rule, the first phase lasts about a day and the second two or three days.

Phase One The first day of any fast is generally marked by pangs of hunger. But don't worry; these are not signs that your body needs food but that your digestive system, accustomed to working on a regular schedule, is simply clicking on and off at the appropriate times. When the hunger pangs strike, try taking several mouthfuls of water; this may effectively deal with the uncomfortable sensations. Besides, you should be drinking at least two quarts of water a day throughout the entire fast.

Phase Two   If you have had recognizable symptoms which you are trying to identify as being related to a sensitivity—such as listlessness, sleeplessness or anxiety—the symptoms may begin to intensify within the first twenty-four hours. This happens because your body is entering a period of withdrawal, when it craves the substance to which it has become sensitive.

In addition, your symptoms may become exaggerated as a result of the release of toxic substances that have been stored in your body. We accumulate toxins every day. The air we breathe is polluted; much of our food as well as the food of the animals we eat has been sprayed with pesticides and other toxic chemicals; many toxic pollutants are dumped into our rivers and oceans and find their way into our bodies via the seafood we eat; and in many parts of the country, a variety of toxic and nontoxic chemicals are added to our drinking water. It is almost impossible, in fact, to live in this culture and avoid being bombarded by toxic substances.

Our bodies have ways of combating some of this toxicity. The liver, for example, acts as a filter, removing toxic materials from the bloodstream, detoxifying them (through a series of chemical reactions), and eliminating them from the body. Our bodies can also handle these toxic substances by storing them in bone or fat.

During a fast, because your body does not have to digest food and deal with the resultant waste products, it has an opportunity to get rid of stored toxic materials through the action of the liver, intestines, lungs, kidneys and skin. As the toxins leave their storage places to be excreted from your body, some may enter the bloodstream, causing a temporary worsening of the condition. New symptoms such as headaches, dizziness, tiredness, and the weak and achy sensations that often accompany the flu may appear.

When toxic symptoms do occur, it is often possible to minimize or even prevent them, one of the most rapid and effective ways being through an enema. During a fast, it is common for bowel movements to cease occurring spontaneously, since there is no food to stimulate the emptying reflex of the bowel. At the same time, however, toxins are being released and need to be eliminated. Without bowel movements, a major avenue of elimination is blocked. Daily enemas overcome this problem and thus are helpful elements of the fast.

The skin is also a major organ of elimination, so it is natural that, along with the mouth, it may start to smell a bit foul when toxic materials are being eliminated. In addition, even the urine and stool may smell differently. These odors are normal side effects as the body eliminates wastes quickly and efficiently.

If your breath turns foul, you may brush your teeth, tongue and gums, but only with a toothbrush that is free of toothpaste. Most toothpastes, like many other commercial products, have a variety of artificial ingredients, including artificial colors and flavorings. If any chemicals to which you happen to be sensitive are part of the paste, you will ingest toxic substances that can cause your symptoms to worsen.

If your skin smells strange, shower frequently. You can also brush your whole body with a dry, stiff, natural-bristled brush, a technique that not only feels wonderful, but rubs off the external layer of dead skin cells—the layer that has accumulated many of the toxic materials. Afterwards, shower away the residue.

Walking in fresh air or other forms of exercise also help the body, particularly the lungs, to eliminate toxic materials; drinking lots of water helps to flush toxins out through the kidneys. The more toxins you eliminate from your body, the better you will feel.

In some instances—and despite careful attention to these measures—you may still experience the discomfort of withdrawal and detoxification. But even if you do nothing to get rid of the symptoms, they will probably disappear in a day or two. However, there are a number of things that can be done to alleviate the discomfort. For instance, you can take a combination of vitamin C and vitamin B-6, or a mixture of sodium and potassium bicarbonate. (For specifics, see pages 109–110.) However, you should check with the medical professional supervising your fast before using either of these measures.

Another way to ease the discomfort is to drink some juice during the period of detoxification. The ingestion of juices—which, however, strictly speaking, breaks the fast—slows down the release of some toxins, and the rich vitamin and mineral content of the juices helps to neutralize others. The major disadvantage is that if you are sensitive to the juice you decide to drink, your symptoms may increase. If you do decide to drink juice, choose one to which you are not likely to be sensitive—that is, one you do not drink regularly. It is best to prepare the juice from raw fruit or vegetables containing no added chemicals. Drink it while it is still very fresh, within five to ten minutes of preparation.

Every individual reacts differently to physical changes in his or her environment, and a fast is a major physical change. Some people feel no different while they are fasting; others feel an increased sense of well-being; still others, as we have mentioned, experience initial discomfort and may continue to feel flulike, achy symptoms well into the third day.

The discomfort is, we repeat, temporary. But you may be so uncomfortable that you want to end your fast; the combination of intensified withdrawal symptoms and the body's reaction to the process of elimination of toxic materials may seem too much for you. In addition, the two can easily be confused. The important thing to remember is that the discomfort can actually be a good thing. In the case of withdrawal, it indicates that you probably do have a definite sensitivity; otherwise you would not feel the discomfort. In the case of detoxification, you are literally revitalizing your body, ridding it of elements that over the years have only slowed you down.

We have personally supervised hundreds of fasts. In almost every case we have been able to overcome or to control sufficiently the discomforts so that the fast could be completed. Less than half a dozen times have we found it necessary to terminate it prematurely. However, it is important to keep in mind that ending the fast is always an available option. When you resume eating, the symptoms of withdrawal and detoxification will generally stop. Relief is, in fact, only as far away as eating some food.

Phase Three   For most people, the third phase begins somewhere around the third or fourth day. It is during this phase that symptoms disappear and a feeling of well-being sets in. However, if the symptoms of withdrawal and toxicity still bother you, you may want to continue for a few more days, in which case you should consult your doctor. (Remember, however, that in some severe chronic cases it may take as many as ten days of fasting to reach the turning point.)

If you do continue to experience discomfort, there are several possible explanations. The problem of toxicity could be greater than you imagined; your system may not be eliminating the wastes quickly enough; your period of withdrawal may be more extensive than average; your symptoms may not be related to a sensitivity at all; you may be sensitive to the juices you have been drinking, or even to the water that has been your only source of sustenance; or your sensitivity may be to something other than food. As we pointed out previously, chemicals in our atmosphere can affect us as strongly as foods and can cause similar problems. If by the fourth or fifth day your symptoms have not yet begun to subside, you should begin to suspect that something in the environment—from gasoline fumes to dust—could be causing your problem.

WHAT A FAST CAN TELL YOU

Although the function of a diagnostic fast is primarily to prepare you for deliberate food testing, it may offer clues to your condition.

1. *If you feel the same throughout the fast with no change in your symptoms:* You may have (a) no sensitivity; (b) a sensitivity that is probably not related to food; or (c) a set of reactions so severe that the symptoms will not clear up after four days of fasting. The fact that you might not have a sensitivity does not mean, however, that fasting was a waste of time. On the contrary, it has given you

a chance to detoxify your body, which in itself is generally a healthful experience.

2. *If you get worse during the first few days and then begin to improve:* This is a clear sign of sensitivity. While certain problems can be caused by the higher level of toxicity in your blood (the flulike sensations we discussed before), an increase and then fading of symptoms usually points to withdrawal from some substance to which you are sensitive.

3. *If you get worse and continue to feel bad for the duration of the fast:* Again, the cause could be either the symptoms of withdrawal or high levels of toxicity in the blood. In addition, it may mean that you were slightly undernourished before you began your fast, or that your body was not properly prepared for the many changes it is going through. Discuss the situation with your doctor and get ready to end your fast, or at least to modify it by drinking juices.

Deliberate Food Testing

When the symptoms you experienced at the beginning of the fast are gone, you are ready to start deliberate food testing. It is now time to work out an eating schedule that can help reveal your sensitivities.

Testing a series of foods is not a haphazard proposition; it takes some preparation. So, before you start your testing, make a list of the foods you normally eat, when you eat them, and how frequently. Underline the name of any food that you eat frequently or crave, or that you suspect may be a sensitizing agent. The underlined foods constitute your "suspicious list." The most important foods to test are those you eat most often. Other foods —foods you only eat in restaurants or during a two-week period in the summer, for instance—are not as important as your usual foods. Furthermore, unless you test these special foods soon after you have been extensively exposed to them, the test can give you a false negative reading—a reading that implies that you are not sensitive, when in fact you will be if you eat the food regularly.

This is because your body can lose its sensitivity if it hasn't been exposed to a food for a while.

Most processed foods are actually combinations of other basic foods. Almost all cakes, for example, contain the basic ingredients of flour, eggs, milk and sugar (which may be derived from sugar cane, beets or corn); all pasta contains flour; most commercial sauces contain either flour or corn syrup as a thickener; and all dairy products, of course, contain milk. When the big three—corn, wheat and milk—are tested, dozens of other foods are tested as well.

Different dairy products should be tested separately, since it is possible to be sensitive to some and not to others. The different ways a product is processed may also be a factor in your sensitivity.

On the first day of the testing period, you should confine yourself to foods to which you are probably not sensitive—various fruits and vegetables—rather than the more likely suspects, such as corn, milk and wheat. When you reintroduce the suspicious foods, try to avoid eating them one after the other to minimize the possibility of having numerous consecutive sensitivity reactions. Once you have the list of foods to test and the order in which to test them, follow the principles listed below for deliberate food testing.

1. *As you begin your testing, exercise some restraint.* Just as it is a good idea to ease into the fast, it is best to ease out as well. It is particularly important not to overeat. Remember that your body has gone without food for quite a while. Just as you would not race the engine of a car before it has warmed up, you should give your body time to adjust to eating food again. In addition, you should avoid taking the chance of consuming a large quantity of food to which you might be sensitive.

2. *Reintroduce foods one at a time.* The reason for this is that if you do have a sensitivity reaction, you will know exactly which food caused it.

3. *Make sure you do not inadvertently mix foods.* For example, if you are having broccoli, remember that the butter you might want to melt over it is a milk product or that margarine contains corn oil. Similarly, a fried egg cooked in butter or lard will carry

some of the properties of grease with it, while a boiled egg will consist only of egg.

4. *Space your meals at regular intervals, eating no more often than every three hours.* In most cases, if three hours have passed and you have had no reaction to whatever you have eaten, you can consider that food safe and go on to the next one.

5. *The foods you test should be in the form in which you usually eat them.* Sometimes a food causes a different reaction, depending on whether it is eaten raw or cooked. Therefore, the test foods should be cooked in the usual way; if you eat certain foods (such as carrots) both raw and cooked, test them both ways.

6. *Be aware that you may react differently to organic and nonorganic foods.* There are foods to which you may have a reaction but to which you may not actually be sensitive: you may be sensitive to elements added to the foods, such as chemicals routinely used in spraying them, or preservatives with which they are combined. Should you seem to be sensitive to a nonorganic food, you may wish to test that same food grown organically. If your sensitivity is to the additive, you should not react to the organic food.

(Be aware, however, that additives may still exist in so-called organic foods. Not all food sold as organic has actually been organically grown. Since the latter generally costs more than nonorganic food, there is an extra profit to be made in labeling food organic when it is not. Often the shopkeeper who sells you the food in good faith is as much a victim of the fraud as you are.)

Note that if you react to many different foods, it is quite possible that you may be sensitive to some chemical or class of chemicals added to them.

7. *If you are a smoker, remember to test cigarettes.* You should have given up smoking as well as eating during the fasting and deliberate food testing. Don't forget to test cigarettes, cigars, and other tobacco products. As with foods, test tobaccos separately.

8. *Be aware that a sensitivity reaction may not occur the first time you eat a food.* If the results of the first test are negative and you are pretty sure that a certain food is giving you trouble, don't hesitate to test the food again at a different time.

9. *Complete the testing within ten days.* For approximately ten days after the fast you will actually be more sensitive to those foods that have been bothering you than you were before, because fasting can unmask hidden food sensitivities. However, beyond this point you may start to lose your sensitivity to foods from which you are continuing to abstain. (For additional information, see Chapter Eight.)

MRS. D AND THE SANDMAN

A good example of this increased sensitivity can be seen in the case of Mrs. D. This pleasant fifty-year-old woman came to see us because her husband of twenty-five years was insisting on a divorce.

Mrs. D explained that for the previous twenty years she had been unable to stay awake for more than an hour or so past supper. She couldn't understand this overwhelming weariness which had become an integral, though unwelcome, part of her life. Even though she had tried many suggestions for keeping awake, none had proved successful. Her husband, who wanted her to share his leisure time, was tremendously resentful of her inability to stay awake in the evenings. After twenty years he had had enough; now that their children were old enough to be on their own, he wanted out of the marriage.

Although Mrs. D loved her husband, she agreed to the divorce, since she saw no hope of ever overcoming the sleep attacks. She came to us for counseling on how to deal with the trauma of divorce. Although we made it clear that we were willing to work with her in the manner she requested, we mentioned the possibility of a brain sensitivity. She was skeptical when we suggested that she begin a fast; but since she was a few pounds overweight anyway, she decided to try it, feeling that the fast would at least help her to lose the excess weight.

She was quite surprised when, on the evening of the third day of the fast, she was able to stay awake late into the night. From that point on, wakefulness became the rule rather than the exception. Her skepticism disappeared, and she was eager to begin testing. In her case, discovering the offending foods proved very easy. Her husband was a meat-and-potatoes man; every night she and her husband ate some form of meat and potatoes.

Mrs. D chose to test the meat first. After having eaten no meat for six days, she then ate a huge, juicy hamburger. It hit her system like a freight train. She ate the hamburger at 1 P.M.; by 1:30 P.M. she was fast asleep. Mrs. D remained asleep for the rest of that day, that evening, and well into the next morning. She stopped eating meat and had no further trouble staying awake. Thus ended her psychiatric treatment; when we last heard from her, she was still married.

This case is a dramatic example of what can happen if breaking the fast is not handled as carefully as the fasting itself. With the body detoxified and literally devoid of food, the first few things that enter the system have power far beyond their normal capacities. So treat your sensitivities carefully. Exercise caution if you engage in activities that require alertness (such as driving a car). Don't break your fast with foods you suspect. And if you can help it, don't eat two types of suspected foods back to back.

If you do experience a reaction to a certain food, and that reaction mimics symptoms you suffered before the fast, you know you are dealing with brain sensitivity. But just because you have discovered one food to which you are sensitive doesn't mean you should stop testing the other foods on your list. Sensitivity to more than one food is the rule rather than the exception.

Because any reaction you experience will interfere with your ability to discern the effects of other foods, stop eating until the reaction wears off. If you feel you must eat, eat only those foods that your testing has proved safe. Only when the effects of your sensitivity have completely worn off should you continue testing other foods.

If you do have a bad reaction to a food, you can also use the methods noted in Chapter Eight for stopping a sensitivity reaction.

Deliberate Food Testing Without Fasting (Elimination Testing)

When testing for brain sensitivities, it is preferable to fast completely rather than to resort to the elimination of individual foods without a fast. Even if you are fairly certain that you are sensitive, it may be difficult to predict exactly which foods are the offending agents. Eliminating suspicious foods for five to ten days and testing a whole series of foods can drag the procedure out for months. More important, testing in this manner can be misleading, because a single symptom like a headache or listlessness may be caused by several different foods independently. For example, you may suspect that your listlessness is due to a milk sensitivity. But when you eliminate milk and milk products from your diet, you notice no change in your symptoms. As a result, you may conclude that milk had nothing to do with your listlessness, an assumption not necessarily correct, since you actually may be sensitive to two or more foods—such as milk, wheat and corn— all of which can be contributing to your listlessness. If you continue to eat wheat and corn and eliminate milk, your symptoms will continue unchanged. Without a complete fast you may not hit upon the exact combination of foods that has caused your listlessness.

Nevertheless, when a complete fast is either impractical or contraindicated, it is often possible to test for sensitivities through a process of eliminating specific foods or food groups for five to ten days before reintroducing them. To increase the accuracy of the test, keep in mind the following points:

1. If there are several foods to which you suspect you are sensitive, eliminate as many at the same time as is practical.

2. Foods that should be most suspect are those you crave. Other suspicious foods are your favorites and those you eat often (daily or several times a week).

3. The three foods most often involved in brain sensitivities are, as we have mentioned, milk, wheat and corn. Those foods would be the best bet for testing, statistically speaking; but of course not every individual will fall into this statistical grouping.

4. Eliminate all suspicious foods for a five- to ten-day period before you begin testing.

5. During the elimination period eat foods that you generally do not eat often, since they are less likely to be sensitizing agents.

6. When eliminating a food, be sure to also eliminate any derivatives of that food. If, for example, you are testing wheat, it is not enough to avoid bread, pasta and crackers; be sure to read the labels on all packaged foods to make sure that none of them contain wheat.

7. When eliminating one food, try to eliminate other foods in the same family as well. Often, there is a cross-sensitivity among such foods. This means that if you are sensitive to potatoes, you may also be sensitive to other foods in the same food family, such as tomatoes, eggplant, paprika and all peppers except black pepper. (See Appendix 2 for a list of food families.)

8. During both the elimination and testing periods, eliminate as many food additives as you possibly can.

During the elimination period, check to see if your symptoms worsen during the initial withdrawal phase (a good prognostic sign) and improve in the latter phase. If neither of these reactions is observed and the symptoms remain essentially unchanged, either your symptoms are not related to a food sensitivity; the foods you are testing are safe foods; or this form of testing is not working, and another form should be tried.

On the other hand, if as a result of this test you do notice a marked improvement, or if the symptoms disappear completely, you should proceed with the second half of the test: the introduction of the eliminated foods one at a time.

Without a complete fast your body may not be as highly sensitive to the reintroduction of foods as it would otherwise be. Therefore, it may be necessary to continue eating each reintroduced food for a few days to determine whether it is safe. Continue this procedure until each of the eliminated foods has been tested. If a reintroduced food brings back the symptoms either soon after its eating or anytime during the week, immediately discontinue that food and wait for the symptoms to subside. If you find that the elimination of a food is associated with an improvement in specific symptoms and that the reintroduction of that food is associated with a return of those same symptoms, you have established the existence of a sensitivity.

Characteristics of Fasting and Deliberate Food Testing

ADVANTAGES

1. It is the most accurate and reliable of the diagnostic tests.
2. The testing itself eliminates the symptoms.
3. The process of reintroducing foods elicits the symptoms, offering dramatic proof of the relationship between the food and the symptoms.
4. The test is free.
5. The test can be performed at home (although it is best done under medical supervision).
6. Fasting also detoxifies the body.
7. Fasting increases susceptibility to sensitivities and therefore makes easier the identification of offending foods. For the same reason, it can unmask hidden sensitivities.
8. It is generally easier to give up an offending food after having avoided it for the duration of the fast.

DISADVANTAGES

1. The idea of fasting is distasteful to many people.
2. An initial period of hunger can cause discomfort, as can symptoms due to withdrawal and detoxification.
3. Fasting and deliberate food testing detect sensitivity to foods, but cannot be used to detect sensitivity to chemicals.
4. Because fasting makes one more susceptible to offending foods, it may elicit a stronger than usual reaction to the reintroduction of that food. That reaction may be severe enough to disrupt normal activities temporarily.

5. Enemas are an important part of the fasting process.
6. Smoking is forbidden during the test.

Characteristics of Elimination Testing

ADVANTAGES

1. The test avoids a total fast.
2. In the process of testing, symptoms are eliminated.
3. Reintroducing foods revives the symptoms, offering dramatic proof of the relationship between the food and the symptoms.
4. There is no expense involved.
5. The test can be performed at home.
6. It is generally easier to give up an offending food after having avoided it for the duration of the fast.
7. Enemas are not required, because no detoxification occurs and bowel movements are not inhibited.

DISADVANTAGES

1. The test is not always as accurate as testing after a fast.
2. Withdrawal symptoms can still occur.
3. The test can only detect sensitivity to foods; it cannot be used to detect sensitivity to chemicals.
4. You must stop smoking during the elimination period.

FOUR:
The Coca Pulse Test

Hundreds of years ago in India, word of the skills of a certain young physician began to spread. The man had a fantastic ability to heal the sick; but, more important, his diagnostic skills were so great that it was said he could identify diseases merely by examining a patient's pulse. One prince who considered himself something of a scientist doubted the rumors; he demanded that the physician be brought before him.

When the man appeared, the prince began to question him. "I have heard," he said, "that you can diagnose any illness simply by taking an individual's pulse." The physician nodded. "I have also heard that your skills are so advanced that you have been known to make accurate diagnoses merely by feeling the beat of the heart through a length of string tied around the wrist." Again the physician nodded.

"We doubt you," said the prince, "and we would like some proof of these purported skills. If you succeed, anything in our principality is yours for the asking. If you fail, you will die."

The physician agreed to the terms of the test and was led into a bare room sectioned in two by a thick blanket. Through the blanket protruded the end of a piece of string.

"Now we shall attach the other end to your patient," said the prince. And he went around the blanket and tied the string around the tibial pulse of a hidden cow.

The physician picked up his end of the string and closed his eyes in concentration. He held the string loosely in his hand, remaining still for a long time. Finally he dropped the string and walked over to the prince.

"Well," asked the prince, "have you made your diagnosis?"

"I have," said the physician, "and I have determined that there is nothing wrong with this patient that a bale of grass wouldn't cure."

This story is a myth, of course, but it indicates the historical importance of the pulse in diagnosis. Before this age of technological sophistication, reading the pulse was one of the more valuable tools available to physicians; for it provided a pathway to the internal workings of the body, a keyhole through which the integrity of the heart and other organs could be studied. In Eastern medicine, testing the pulse is still a major aid in diagnosis; traditional acupuncturists test it at twelve different points for clues to the health of nearly every body organ and function.

In the West, however, examination of the pulse has become less important as an indicator of subtle change. Yet even as traditional medicine has been deemphasizing the use of the pulse for diagnostic purposes, some doctors have been discovering new uses for it. In the 1930s Dr. Arthur Coca, for example, discovered that testing the pulse was a simple yet effective way to determine the existence of sensitivities to foods, inhalants and chemicals. His wife had been hospitalized following an attack of angina pectoris (heart pain). Mrs. Coca's condition was severe. She had been incapacitated for three years, and two heart specialists had predicted that she didn't have much longer to live. While visiting her in the hospital, Dr. Coca noted that a pulse rate of 180 beats per minute had been recorded on her chart. When he asked her about this extremely rapid rate, she remarked that she had noticed that her pulse sometimes tended to race after meals. Surprised, Dr. Coca suggested that she eat one food at a time and have her pulse checked after each meal. The Cocas discovered that potatoes shot Mrs. Coca's pulse up to that incredible 180 beats per minute; certain other foods also tended to speed it up, but not so much. Mrs. Coca stopped eating those particular foods.

More than twenty years later Mrs. Coca was not only alive, but free from heart pain as long as she avoided the foods that increased her pulse rate. This alone would have been enough of a blessing, but the Cocas found that other ailments she had suffered for years—migraines, colitis, attacks of dizziness and fainting, abnormal tiredness, and indigestion—had also disappeared.

Elated, Dr. Coca began to use the pulse test in a similar way with his patients. He quickly learned that many symptoms affecting different parts of the body could be treated successfully as allergies. These problems included various pathologies linked to the brain, from epilepsy to emotional instability, nervousness and depression.

Four factors seemed to indicate the allergic nature of these conditions:

1. The symptoms disappeared when the implicated foods were eliminated from the diet.

2. Many patients suffered from a variety of completely different symptoms, all of which disappeared together when offending foods or chemicals were discontinued.

3. In most cases the symptoms could be brought back if the foods were reintroduced into the diet.

4. Symptoms were accompanied by an increase in the pulse rate.

SEIZURE-FREE B.B.

One of the many cases reported by Dr. Coca was that of a college student, B.B., who suffered from epilepsy as well as headaches, abnormal tiredness, neuralgia and nervousness. Despite the medications he was taking, B.B. had minor seizures every day and major seizures almost as often. The epileptic episodes had, in fact, become so frequent that B.B. had to drop out of college.

Using the pulse test, Dr. Coca found that B.B. reacted to wheat, oranges, pineapples and asparagus. When B.B. avoided these foods, the seizures stopped and he could stop taking medication.

B.B. continued to shun these foods for three months; during that time he remained free of both his seizures and his other

symptoms. Then one evening he deliberately ate some bread, and
the next morning he suffered a major seizure. B.B. returned to his
diet for six months, experiencing no further attacks until one day
he ate spaghetti made from wheat. The following morning he
suffered another major seizure during which he broke a tooth.

Apparently B.B. needed these experiences to convince him
that there was a distinct connection between the seizures and
what he ate. He began to realize that by strict adherence to his
diet he could prevent the epileptic attacks. Only then was he able
to return to college and finish his studies.

Performing the Pulse Test at Home

HOW TO TAKE YOUR PULSE

The pulse test is based on a simple, easy-to-prove premise: your
pulse rate generally accelerates after you eat foods or inhale substances to which you are sensitive. Testing your pulse to uncover
sensitivities is not difficult, but it does require a commitment on
your part to a program of testing and analysis that may take a week
or longer.

Each time the heart beats, it pumps blood into the arteries,
causing an intermittent buildup of pressure. You can feel this
pressure as a pulse whenever you hold your fingers on an artery.
The pulse can be felt in a variety of places, including the neck,
the temple and the ankle. The wrist is most often used.

To feel the pulse in your wrist, rest one hand in your lap
with the palm facing up. Then trace the thumb down to
where the palm meets the wrist and place one or two fingertips of your other hand at that point. By pressing lightly with
your fingertips, you should feel the pulse. If you don't feel the
pulse immediately, try varying the pressure and position of
your fingers.

Your pulse rate is the number of times your heart beats per
minute. In testing for sensitivities, make sure to count the beats
for a full sixty seconds; counting for fifteen seconds and multiply-

ing by four can modify your reading by as many as four or more beats, which for our purposes is a significant difference.

BEFORE YOU BEGIN THE TEST

According to Dr. Coca, the following steps must be undertaken at least two or three days before the testing begins:

1. You *must* stop smoking before and refrain from smoking during the pulse test. Tobacco is a major cause of sensitivities and can distort the results of the test. (You can test your sensitivity to tobacco after you have finished testing foods.)

2. You must keep a written record of your pulse rate, making fourteen separate recordings a day, for at least two or three days before the test. Test your pulse at the following times:

    (a) just after waking up in the morning, but before getting out of bed;

    (b) just before each meal;

    (c) three times after each meal, at half-hour intervals; and

    (d) just before going to sleep.

Each of these fourteen pulse counts should be taken while you are sitting down, except for the first one of the day; it should be taken while you are still lying in bed.

3. Remember to write down each food you eat at each meal. If you eat something like vegetable soup (which is composed of a variety of different foods), be sure to list each ingredient.

4. If you want to eat, drink or chew gum between meals, be sure to wait at least an hour and a half after your last meal so that the snacks won't interfere with your pulse recordings. Snack foods should be treated as separate meals and listed on your chart also, along with the time you ate them. Your pulse should again be tested once before and three times at half-hour intervals after you eat.

Because normal pulse rates can differ significantly from individual to individual, the preparatory steps listed above are crucial. You must determine your own characteristic rates before you can actually begin testing. Your pretest recordings will be used to arrive at three different factors: (a) your lowest pulse rate each day; (b) your highest pulse rate each day; and (c) the difference each day between your lowest and highest rates (your pulse differential).

As you evaluate these pretest recordings, keep the following guidelines in mind:

1. Under normal conditions the pulse rate is fairly stable, but of course charged emotional situations and physical exercise can cause it to speed up.

2. Your lowest pulse rate during the day usually occurs before you arise in the morning. However, if you are sensitive to something in your bedroom (a feather pillow; dust in your bedding), or even to food you ate the night before, the first rate you record may well be higher than some of the later ones.

3. If your pulse differential is greater than 12 during any single day—if, for example, your high is 82 and your low rate is 69—you may have a sensitivity to something you ate that day; if your differential is greater than 16—e.g., high of 88, low of 66—you most likely have a sensitivity; and if your pulse differential does not exceed 12 in any of the three pretest days, you are probably not sensitive to any of the foods you ate on those days.

4. If your daily high pulse varies by more than two beats from day to day, you most likely have a sensitivity. On the other hand, if your high pulse rate remains consistently within one or two beats from day to day, you have probably not eaten anything to which you are sensitive.

5. In the absence of an obvious cause (such as infection, sunburn, strenuous physical or emotional activity), a large increase over your characteristic pulse at any one recording can usually be traced to a sensitivity reaction.

THE PULSE TEST

The record you have established during the three pretest days now makes it possible to evaluate individual foods. To begin your testing, make a list of the foods you wish to evaluate. Be sure to include any food that you suspect may be causing a sensitivity reaction, as well as the foods you eat regularly. If your pretest information has indicated a probable sensitivity, use it to zero in on possible culprits. (For example, if your pulse rate rose significantly after you ate a meal that included beef, potatoes, bread and broccoli, be sure to include these foods in your testing.) An increase in your pulse rate in the morning before you have eaten should lead you to suspect a chemical or inhalant sensitivity, while an increase after a specific meal tends to implicate one or more of the foods eaten at that meal.

A minimum of two days is usually required to complete the testing. To use the test effectively, follow this procedure:

1. When you wake up, record your pulse as you did during the pretest period.

2. Throughout the rest of the day, eat a small amount of a different food each hour.

3. Count your pulse just before eating and a half hour after eating each food, and record the results.

4. If your pulse rate increases after you eat a food, wait until your pulse returns to normal before testing another food. Although it isn't common, it's possible for a reaction (increased pulse rate) to last several hours. At times this reaction may be erratic; for example, a higher rate may settle down, only to increase again. This pattern may recur several times before the pulse steadies. Therefore, after an increased rate, allow your pulse to normalize for at least one hour before testing the next food.

5. If you are sensitive to a certain food but have not eaten it for a few weeks, you may find no increase in pulse rate during your first test. Therefore, if you test a food you haven't eaten in a while, test it a second time two or three days later.

6. You can test chemicals and inhalants in a similar way. Expose yourself to whatever chemical you choose to test exactly as you would be exposed to it under normal circumstances. For example, if you suspect you react to the gas from your stove, stand near the stove for at least five minutes while the burners are on, and breathe normally. (It is best not to have food on the burners while you are doing this, since fumes from the food may be a source of sensitivity.) To test auto exhaust, stand outside near traffic; to test

perfume, either put some on or open the bottle and inhale its fumes for a minute; to test house dust, vacuum and/or dust your house as usual; to test a pet cat or dog, hold the animal close to your nose for a few minutes and breathe normally. Record your pulse just before, just after and a half hour after the test. Note also whether any symptoms develop during or shortly after the test.

Interpreting the Test

Use the following rules as guidelines in interpreting the information accumulated from the pulse test. Note that these are not rigid rules; pulse rates and discrepancies vary from individual to individual, and exceptions do exist.

1. If a food that you eat frequently does not cause your pulse rate to increase at least six beats above your normal high pulse rate, that food is probably nonallergenic.

2. If a food causes your pulse to increase six or more beats above your normal high rate, it is most likely a sensitizing agent.

3. A pulse count above 84 beats per minute unaccounted for by other known factors generally indicates an allergy either to the test material or to something in the environment.

4. If your pulse differential remains high no matter what you eat, you are sensitive either to almost all the foods you have tested or to something you are constantly inhaling.

5. Pulse reactions to inhaled allergens usually do not last so long and are not so severe as those to food allergens.

6. An increase in your pulse rate of less than six beats per minute during a test is usually due to an inhalant.

7. If, after you have completed your testing of foods and inhalants, you go back to smoking and decide to test it as well, note that if you are sensitive, your pulse will usually increase within fifteen minutes from the time you began to smoke.

Characteristics of the Pulse Test

ADVANTAGES

1. Pulse testing is an accurate, objective method of uncovering sensitivities.
2. It can be used to test foods, inhalants and chemicals.
3. It is safe and free.
4. It can be performed at home.

DISADVANTAGES

1. You may get withdrawal symptoms during the testing.
2. The test requires time and concentration: you must remember to make multiple recordings for at least a week.
3. For the test to be accurate, you must stop smoking.
4. You must curtail your snacking, gum chewing, etc., for the duration of the test.
5. Other external factors, such as physical or emotional activities or exposure to extraneous chemicals during the testing, may alter the accuracy.

FIVE:
Kinesiologic Testing

Kinesiologic testing is the simplest, yet to most people the most foreign, of the methods to test brain sensitivities at home. While the idea of fasting and pulse taking as tests for sensitivities may seem unusual, at least the concepts involved are familiar. Kinesiologic testing, on the other hand, introduces a concept unfamiliar to most of us; in fact, the test itself may appear to smack of magic or trickery. We ourselves had trouble believing it when we first saw it demonstrated, but our trust has grown slowly over the years as kinesiologic testing has proved valid time and time again.

To understand this new concept, let's consider a simple analogy. Electricity is a phenomenon we take utterly for granted. Although electrical current is invisible to the naked eye, we don't question what is happening; we have grown up with electricity, have lived with it all our lives; a world without electrical appliances would seem very strange to us now.

To someone who has never encountered it, however, the whole idea must seem like magic, difficult to believe. An explanation of electricity as "a swift flow of invisible particles" would probably only confuse the issue and might elicit the perfectly logical question: "How can you tell me these things are moving when you can't see them?"

Modern science's experience with the human body follows a similar course. Although we have mapped many of the body's larger structures, and although we have a fairly good understanding of many of the systems that make it work, there are probably parts and pathways we have not even discovered, much less begun to understand.

Kinesiologic testing, one of the methods of diagnosing brain sensitivity, fits into the category of what is still unknown. We have proved that it works, and you can prove it to yourself. But as to why and how it works, we can only guess.

As it applies to the determination of brain sensitivity, kinesiologic testing is basically the test of a muscle's strength before and after an external force has influenced the body. If the muscle's strength remains the same, the influence has been either neutral or positive; if its strength decreases, the influence has been negative.

Kinesiologic testing is part of an overall branch of the healing arts known as applied kinesiology. Developed by Dr. George Goodheart, applied kinesiology is based on the concept that the body itself knows what is wrong with it and what is necessary to make it well. Most of us have lost contact with the wisdom residing in our own bodies. The impact of our commercialized, industrialized society has left us so out of touch with ourselves that we no longer consciously understand what our bodies do and do not need to remain healthy. In a sense, we have stopped listening to ourselves. But whether we are conscious of our bodies' signals or not, they do exist and can be tapped.

By testing the reaction of one muscle to, let's say, a specific food, we are once again allowing the body to speak for itself. Kinesiologic testing allows us to open the lines of communication by concentrating on a single, specific reaction.

How to Test Kinesiologically

Kinesiologic testing requires two people: the person doing the testing and the person being tested. Because testing the strength of an individual's muscle might very well degenerate into a contest of muscular strength, let us emphasize from the beginning that what we are discussing has nothing to do with arm wrestling but is a dual effort to form a preliminary diagnosis.

Any muscle of the body that is normal, strong and intact can be used for the testing. We prefer using the arm because it is convenient and easy to test.

First, test the muscle normally. Hold your arm out in front of you or to the side, with the palm facing down. Then have the person testing you face you and either grasp your wrist or place one or more fingers on it. As you try to resist, have that person push down quickly and firmly, without jerking, in an effort to force your arm to your side. Together, you should be able to establish approximately how much resistance you can muster.

Now you have an idea of your normal strength. To test a food for brain sensitivity, chew a small mouthful and place it under your tongue. If it is liquid, mix it with some saliva and hold it under your tongue. In neither case should you swallow the food. While the food is still in contact with your tongue, test the muscle again. If it remains as strong as before you began your testing, you are probably not sensitive to the food. If your arm has weakened —and often it weakens significantly—you are probably sensitive to the food. Then proceed to test one food after another, giving yourself a few moments between tests. Make sure you don't swallow the foods to which the test indicated you had a sensitivity; spit them out and rinse your mouth carefully before testing a new food. Leaving the residue in your mouth will interfere with the foods you test later; and, if you do swallow those foods, they can continue to affect the rest of your testing once they have been absorbed into the bloodstream.

To test for sensitivities to inhalants or chemicals, use the same basic procedure. But instead of placing the material to be tested into your mouth, inhale it. In other words, first test the muscle for its normal strength. Then inhale the substance you are interested in testing and retest the muscle strength. A weakened muscle indicates that you are probably sensitive to that substance.

That is the entire test. Does it seem a little hard to believe? If so, try a simple kinesiologic test on a few friends, using wheat, corn, milk, sugar and coffee. Since brain sensitivities may be found in most people, and since these five substances frequently elicit symptoms, there is a very good chance that a sensitivity to one or more of them will show up in several of the people you test.

Because it takes very little time to test any one food, kinesiologic testing is a quick, simple way to go through a variety of foods in a short period. To check whether a food is still affecting your system after you have washed it out of your mouth, simply test the arm (or whatever other muscle you are using) again; if the strength of the muscle has returned to normal, you are ready to continue testing.

How It Works

Kinesiologic testing works; you can prove it to yourself. But for most people, that is not good enough; they also want to know *how* it works.

Modern medicine has no reliable explanation for what is going on when your arm muscle weakens because of a bit of food in your mouth. It can, however, offer a few reasonable hypotheses. In addition, other systems of medicine have their own explanations of why kinesiologic testing works so well. Let's look at three schools of thought.

THE REFLEX HYPOTHESIS

This hypothesis, which is in line with the thinking of modern medicine, considers that there is actually a reflex action—called a neurolingual (brain-tongue) reflex—that causes the muscles to react so quickly to food in the mouth.

The neurolingual reflex is analogous to the knee-jerk reflex. The doctor taps your knee to see whether he can make your leg jump. What is being tested has very little to do with either the knee or the foot, but with a reflex arc that extends from the knee to the spine, and from the spine to the muscles in the leg, which are contracted when the arc is stimulated. That same test allows the doctor to evaluate the integrity of the spine-brain connection as well. When the doctor taps your knee, he is actually stimulating a nerve. That nerve sends a message to the spinal cord, which hooks up the message with another nerve returning to the muscles in your leg. It is that second nerve which causes your leg to jerk. As for the brain, it normally has an inhibitory effect on the strength of any reflex, literally closing down on some of the power of the impulse returning to the leg. So, by testing that one reflex in the leg, your doctor is able to determine, first, whether the reflex arc from your leg to your spine is intact; and second, whether the pathways from your spine to your brain are sound.

The reflex hypothesis holds that the mouth-arm reaction works in the same way. When you are testing, you are actually finding out what happens in the communication between the tongue and the brain at the moment food enters your mouth. When the food touches your tongue, a message is sent to your brain, which then monitors its quality (and determines whether it is good or bad for you) and sends a message to your muscle.

THE NEUROVASCULAR HYPOTHESIS

A variation of the reflex hypothesis points out that material placed under the tongue can be absorbed very rapidly into the body. One example of this is the relationship between nitroglycerin and angina pectoris. Often, people with heart disease take nitroglycerin to relieve chest pain. If the pain is severe, they are told to put the nitroglycerin under the tongue; they are not to swallow it. The reason is that angina pectoris requires rapid relief; not only is the pain severe, but it may foreshadow a heart attack. Short of injecting the drug into a vein or inhaling it (getting it to the lungs and thereby into the bloodstream almost immediately), the fastest way to send a drug to the heart is to put it under the tongue, from which it quickly enters the bloodstream. If it were swallowed, the same drug might require long minutes, even hours, of digestion before it could reach the circulatory system and begin to work. When chewed food is placed under the tongue, parts of it, like the nitroglycerin, can rapidly enter the bloodstream and reach the brain. The brain may then send impulses via nerves to the muscles, resulting in a weakening or strengthening of the musculature.

THE CONCEPT OF ENERGY FLOW

It is important to recognize that, as effective as Western medicine has proved to be, other concepts of medical treatment have existed for at least as long and have also been shown to be effective.

There are many similarities between the Eastern and Western schools of medical thought. But one major difference is the East's belief in a principle that the West neglects: the hypothesis that "life energy" circulates through the body. Different cultures have different names for this energy. The Indians call it "Prana"; the Chinese call it "Chi"; the Japanese call it "Ki." But it all adds up to the same thing: a form of energy, necessary for life and as yet undiscovered by modern physics, that flows through the body in much the same way as blood, using precise channels and pathways. But whereas the pathways of blood-flow—veins, arteries, capillaries—are major anatomical structures that can be traced and physically drawn, the pathways of energy-flow—called meridians—have never actually been seen anatomically. As a result, despite thousands of years of clinical experience in the East, practitioners of medicine in the West question their existence.

The Eastern concept of illness and health is closely tied to the concept of the flow of this life energy. Health is seen as a state in which a balanced flow of energy exists, both in the organism and between the organism and its environment; and illness is a result of an imbalance in the flow of this energy—a result of too much or too little energy flowing to one part of the body or between the organism and its environment. If the imbalance is allowed to go uncorrected, it ultimately affects the body, leading to recognizable symptoms or disease. Correcting the energy imbalance (as acupuncture attempts to do) can promote healing and lead to a restoration of health. There is, however, a point of no return—a point at which, if the energy is allowed to remain out of balance, the resultant physical damage can become so severe that rebalancing the energy flow may no longer be enough.

This concept of life energy can offer us a new and interesting explanation for what goes on when we test for brain sensitivities kinesiologically. In Eastern philosophy, life energy is thought to be present in all matter; living matter is distinguished from non-living matter mainly by the former's greater concentration of energy. As a result, whenever two bodies approach, their energies influence each other, just as the poles of two magnets attract or repel each other when they are brought close together. Thus, in kinesiologic testing, when you place food in your mouth, the energy of that food interacts with the energy of your body. When pressure is exerted on your arm, you are actually measuring the effect of this interaction on your muscle strength. A food to which you are sensitive causes a rapid but temporary weakening of your muscle, a result of the sudden imbalance imposed on your energy system.

This hypothesis is not so foreign to our way of thinking as it might first appear. A basic premise in physics is that all matter, living and nonliving, is composed of atoms. Atoms, in turn, are composed of electrons whirling around a central nucleus. Their activity creates an electromagnetic energy field around each atom. Thus, all matter is surrounded by energy fields that can interact with one another.

It is still a mystery whether electromagnetic fields, life energy forces, neurovascular pathways, neurolingual reflexes, or some as yet undiscovered mechanism is responsible for the results noted in kinesiologic testing. There is no mystery, however, as to whether or not kinesiologic testing can be used as an effective method of determining sensitivity to foods, inhalants and chemicals when it is done properly and its limitations are understood.

Kinesiologic testing is a very delicate procedure, in that anything that affects the brain can also affect the muscle strength. The brain, of course, is affected by both external and internal stimuli, from those picked up by your five senses to physical reactions within your body and thoughts within your mind. Since any of these stimuli are capable of weakening or strengthening a muscle, it is important that you eliminate or keep constant as many of them as you can while you perform your testing. You can achieve the most reliable results when your surroundings are stable and your mind is relaxed.

Note that in addition to these factors, your test results can be influenced by the time of day the test is conducted. We treated a man who was sensitive to rice and who would feel sleepy after eating it—but only at lunchtime. At dinnertime, when the stresses and hassles of the day had subsided, he would not become sleepy as a result of eating rice. His kinesiologic tests paralleled the pattern in his life: eating rice at noon caused a weakening of the arm, while eating it in the evening had little or no effect on his muscle strength.

Just for Fun . . . Or Is It?

We have noted that muscle testing is influenced not just by foods, chemicals and inhalants, but by a host of other factors as well. When the test is done properly, it can often be used to assess the influence of a whole range of these stimuli on your well-being.

If this sounds strange, you can try it out yourself. The following experiments initially suggested to us by Dr. John Diamond, the founder of behavioral kinesiology, can serve as a starting point. Simply test each stimulus as you previously tested foods, and decide whether your body reacts.

1. *Music.* Test the effects of different types of music, from the Beatles and the Rolling Stones to Bach and Beethoven. Then test the effects of the same kinds of music at different levels of loudness.

2. *Voices.* Test the effects of different people's voices. You can use live voices as well as those recorded on tape or broadcast over radio or TV.

3. *Television.* Stand near a TV that is turned off and establish your normal muscle strength. Then turn on the TV and retest your muscle. Do the test at different distances from the TV; if your muscle becomes weak when you are close to the tube, try to

determine a "safe" distance, where your strength returns to normal. Try separate tests with color and black-and-white TVs.

4. *Lighting.* Test the effects of sunlight, fluorescent light and incandescent light.

5. *Jewelry.* Test the effects of different pieces of jewelry. First remove the jewelry and establish your normal muscle strength without it; then put it back on and repeat the test. If you simply try to test the effect while it is on, your body may have established a new equilibrium and adapted to the jewelry. The muscle might then seem normal even though the jewelry might be affecting you.

6. *Clothing.* Test the effects of different fabrics. Note whether there is any difference between clothing made of natural material (cotton, silk, wool) and clothing woven from synthetic fibers (nylon, dacron, polyester). Pay particular attention to clothing that is in direct contact with your body (such as underwear or a hat). As with jewelry, to test the effect of an article of clothing you are wearing, first remove it and establish your normal muscle strength. Then put it back on and retest the muscle.

7. *Thoughts.* Test the effects of different thought patterns. For example, after establishing your normal muscle strength, concentrate on something you hate or dislike intensely. While retaining that thought, test your muscle strength again. Then do the same thing with something or someone you trust, enjoy or love.

8. *Poetry and Prose.* Test the effects of the written word. After establishing your normal strength, read a passage of prose or a verse of poetry. Retest your muscle. Try to compare radically different kinds of writing to determine whether or not certain specific elements affect you.

These eight experiments are only a few examples of countless things you might want to test. You can check out other possibilities as well; things that might have bothered you in the past or that might have made you say, "I don't know why, but I just don't like . . . that painting . . . that piece of furniture . . . that advertisement."

Characteristics of Kinesiologic Testing

ADVANTAGES

1. It can be done at home, whenever you feel you are ready to try it.
2. It is free, requiring only the assistance of one willing friend.
3. It is safe.
4. Results are immediate.
5. It can be used to test chemicals and inhalants (by a "sniff test") as well as foods.
6. It is possible to test many substances in a short period of time.
7. Because the testing can be done very quickly, tests on various foods can be repeated each time you eat.

DISADVANTAGES

1. The test does not reproduce the symptoms.
2. The test does not include the element of treatment (as fasting does).
3. Without complete concentration, you can easily miss small weaknesses, and you may never accurately determine the true normal strength of the arm.
4. Because the tests can follow each other so closely, it is easy to forget to thoroughly wash away any food to which you are sensitive before testing the next food.
5. Because of the variety of internal and external factors that can affect testing, conditions under which the testing is performed must be very consistent; otherwise, the results of your tests may be inaccurate.
6. Since thoughts can also influence the results, your mind must remain free of extraneous thoughts that might interfere with the testing. (It is actually best to keep your mind blank.) The more suggestible you are, the more important this factor.
7. Unless your partner is experienced (and it is almost certain that he or she is not), there is a tendency for kinesiologic testing

to turn into an arm-wrestling contest. If your partner cannot get your arm down, he tends to try harder, to strain to force your arm to your side. As a result, you may both end up with muscle fatigue (which might spoil the test's accuracy), or even with torn or strained muscles. The problem is easy to avoid, of course, if you will simply remember why you are testing. If your arm begins to tire, you can either use a different muscle or adjourn and resume later.

8. The results may not be accurate if the person testing you is considerably weaker than you. For example, if a child tests an adult, even a fifty percent loss of strength might go unnoticed during the test.

SIX:
Four Laboratory Tests

In addition to the tests you can perform at home, there are laboratory tests which can be used to diagnose brain sensitivities. We shall discuss four. All require the supervision of a physician and are usually performed in his office.

Two of the tests—the intradermal provocative test and the sublingual test—require your active participation throughout the testing. The other two—cytotoxic testing and the radio-allergo-sorbant test (RAST)—are blood tests, which means that you have to stay around only until your blood is drawn.

Intradermal Provocative Testing

Intradermal provocative testing bears a vague resemblance to the allergy "scratch" tests usually associated with classical allergies. In the scratch test, the allergist makes a series of ten to twenty tiny scratches along a patient's back or arm and places a small amount of a different allergen—an extract of whatever he suspects the patient is allergic to—in each scratch. (He may instead inject the allergens directly into the skin.) After twenty minutes the allergist examines the scratches for signs of reddening and swelling, indications that the patient is reacting allergically.

The scratch test is effective in determining which inhalants (such as grasses, pollens and molds) are causing common allergic diseases such as hay fever, asthma and eczema. But it is not nearly as effective in uncovering food allergies. Fortunately its close cousin, the intradermal provocative test, is more reliable.

The intradermal provocative test, which is actually a modification of the scratch test, was introduced in the 1930s. At that time allergists had been using the scratch test as an aid in devising vaccines that could help desensitize their patients against the cause of their allergies. Unfortunately, making those vaccines involved a degree of guesswork. But Dr. Herbert Rinkel (who had stumbled onto his own sensitivity to eggs a short time before) found a way to reduce the arbitrariness involved in making up these vaccines.

While other allergists would test for allergies by injecting a single concentration of approximately twenty allergens at different sites, Rinkel worked with only one allergen at a time, injecting as many as nine different concentrations (dilutions) of that allergen, each succeeding one only one-fifth as strong as the one before. He would then examine his patient for changes caused by the different dilutions.

During his experiments Rinkel paid particular attention to the wheals—the small, raised mounds of skin—left by the injections. He noticed that the wheals left by some dilutions didn't change, while others actually grew larger after the injections. This indicated that the body was secreting a fluid into the area—a clear sign of an allergic reaction. The swelling of the wheals increased in proportion to the concentration he was using.

By studying this whealing response, Rinkel was able to come up with a method for determining accurate desensitizing doses, doses that depended no longer on guesswork but on a reading of the exact point at which the wheals began to swell.

The Rinkel Dilution Titration Technique (as it is called) is still used today by some physicians to uncover allergies and to determine desensitizing doses.

Rinkel tried his technique on foods as well as inhalants, but as late as 1959 he was still unsuccessful. It remained up to a colleague of his, Dr. Carleton Lee, to discover how to detect and treat food allergies by modifying Rinkel's method.

INTRADERMAL PROVOCATIVE TESTING FOR FOODS

Dr. Lee found that by injecting certain dilutions of food allergens, he could provoke symptoms such as headaches, lethargy and runny noses in some of his patients. Then he discovered that if he tried different dilutions of the allergen that had provoked the symptoms, one of them could almost invariably turn off—or neutralize—the symptoms immediately.

Lee began to experiment with his new technique, inducing symptoms with one concentration and neutralizing them with the next. It soon became clear that this was something more than a parlor trick, because his patients began to report that when they received a "neutralizing" dose, they could eat the offending food for three or four days without developing any symptoms.

Lee soon found that if a patient entered his office while suffering from symptoms caused by a particular food, he could stop those symptoms within ten minutes simply by injecting a previously determined neutralizing dose. And he also learned that if he injected the same dose prophylactically—that is, *before* the symptoms occurred—he could actually prevent them from surfacing.

These experiments enabled Lee to work out a number of guidelines for determining the neutralizing dose for a food. He described the symptoms that would appear when a dose was too strong or too weak. He suggested that clinicians could actually base their estimates of neutralizing doses on objective observations of changes in the patient (increased pulse rate, change in color, increased sweating) and the subjective responses of the patient himself (headaches, tension, feelings of restlessness or irritability). And, because his conclusions were based on responses to a single food, he recommended testing one dilution of one food at a time, with a ten-minute period of observation between the injections.

In 1965 Dr. Joseph Miller, a classically trained allergist from Mobile, Alabama, began to work with the methods devised by Rinkel and Lee. By combining their concepts and modifying their techniques, he devised an intradermal provocative test that would uncover food sensitivities not only by provoking and neutralizing symptoms, as Lee had done, but by establishing a correlation between the whealing response (the size of the wheals) and the concentration of the neutralizing dose, similar to Rinkel's work with inhalants.

THE NEUTRALIZING DOSE

For every food to which you are sensitive there exists a specific concentration of that food that will not trigger a reaction, but will instead temporarily block the usual symptoms caused by eating that food.

There are no sure explanations of how the neutralizing dose works. Some physicians believe that it may cause the body to release blocking antibodies which can prevent the reaction that normally takes place. Others believe it follows a basic principle of homeopathic medicine—namely, that like heals like. Homeopathic physicians believe that symptoms are actually attempts on the part of the body to heal itself of a disease process. Consequently, when someone becomes ill, a homeopathic approach would be to prescribe a minute dose of a substance that could intensify the symptoms he already has and thus stimulate the body to heal itself.

How does this work in practice? Assume that you have been troubled by headaches. As a result of testing, you find that the headaches are caused by milk sensitivity. You know then that if you avoid milk and milk products, your headaches will probably disappear. However, there is one specific concentration of milk that not only will not produce a headache, but, if taken just before you eat any dairy products, will protect you from the headaches they would usually cause. This specific concentration is called the neutralizing dose. (It is important to realize that there is no universal neutralizing dose. Two people with sensitivities to the same food may require different neutralizing doses of that food, depending on the degree of their sensitivity, their own personal body chemistry, and other factors.)

In a recently reported double-blind study, Dr. Joseph Miller demonstrated the effectiveness of neutralizing doses of food allergens. He first enlisted the aid of eight patients who had been suffering for years with symptoms such as migraine headaches, chronic diarrhea, mouth sores, abdominal cramps, nasal congestion, irritability and fatigue. Using his intradermal technique, Miller prepared a solution for each patient containing neutralizing doses of the offending foods. At the same time a placebo solution was prepared, which looked the same as the active solution but lacked the neutralizing doses. During the experiment, the patients were encouraged to eat all offending foods for which neutralizing doses had been made. For a total of 80 days, broken down into four 20-day periods, these patients injected themselves under the skin once a day. For two of the four periods they injected the solution containing the neutralizing doses; for the other two they used the placebo. Neither the physician nor the patients had any idea which solution was being used during each period.

At the end of the experiment, when the code was broken, the results were dramatic. The symptoms of all eight patients greatly improved when they unknowingly injected the solution containing the neutralizing doses. On the other hand, the symptoms worsened during the periods when the placebo solution was injected.

A statistical analysis of this experiment revealed that results such as these could only occur by chance at the odds of two to a thousand. This indicates a high degree of statistical reliability.

THE TEST

Because the test involves injections of minute amounts of allergens, it must be performed in a physician's office. Once you and your physician have determined which foods should be tested, he will inject a dilution of one food extract and, after ten minutes, measure the wheal it leaves. The size of the wheal and the type of subjective or objective reaction you have (if any) determine the dilution he will inject next.

If there is a reaction, you have a sensitivity to that food. The physician will then continue to inject different dilutions of that same food to determine the correct neutralizing dose.

If, after the first injection, you have no reaction, there are three possible explanations:

1. You are not sensitive to that food.

2. You are sensitive, but the concentration is too weak to cause a reaction.

3. The physician has hit upon the neutralizing dose.

He will then test two more dilutions of the same food. A reaction to either of them will indicate that you are sensitive. No reaction to any of the three will indicate that you are not sensitive.

When you have completed testing all the foods selected and have determined the necessary neutralizing doses, a vaccine of those doses can be made that will often stop or at least will reduce your sensitivity reactions. (See page 109 for more information.)

POSSIBLE DANGERS

When carried out properly, the intradermal provocative test is extremely safe. Just about the only people who should not undergo the test are severe asthmatics (during an attack or shortly thereafter) and persons with a severe cardiovascular condition (involving heart failure). Diabetics have been tested successfully, as have pregnant women.

Characteristics of Intradermal Provocative Testing

ADVANTAGES

1. The intradermal provocative test is an accurate method for determining the presence or absence of food sensitivities.

2. The test embodies a way of determining one form of treatment—the neutralizing dose.

3. Because of the whealing response, the test is effective even when the patient cannot or will not give accurate subjective responses to testing.

4. A modification of the method can be used to test certain environmental chemicals and inhalants, in addition to foods.

5. In addition to creating a whealing response, the test can sometimes reproduce symptoms, which helps to convince the patient of the relationship between the symptoms and the food.

6. The whealing response is relatively unaffected by environmental conditions.

7. For some patients the results of an objective test carry more weight and credibility than those of the more subjective tests.

DISADVANTAGES

1. The method is time-consuming; only a few foods can be tested during each visit.

2. The test is expensive, mainly because of the time, personnel and equipment needed to administer it.

3. Because it requires many separate injections, the test can be slightly uncomfortable. On the other hand, even most children have little trouble getting through it.

4. The possibility exists that the injection of material to which a person is sensitive will provoke a severe reaction. (However, the reaction can usually be controlled.)

5. Since soluble forms of foods are used, only those portions of a food that can be dissolved are capable of being tested. For example, that part of a carrot which cannot be dissolved will not be included in the final concentrate. Although this is generally not a problem, there may be occasions when a patient is sensitive only to the fraction of the carrot that doesn't dissolve. For that person the test will give a false negative reading.

Sublingual Provocative Testing

The laboratory setting for sublingual provocative testing is similar to the one for intradermal provocative testing, and the test has similar concepts behind it. Since nothing is injected, there is no whealing response; but the technician does place soluble extracts of different foods under the tongue and records the patient's reactions.

THE TEST

The test itself is straightforward. Once you and the physician have determined which foods you will test, a quantity (usually about five drops) of a food extract is placed under your tongue and is held there for ten minutes, while you and the examiner search for any symptoms that might appear.

If no reaction occurs after ten minutes, a lower concentration of the same food is tested; after ten more minutes, if still no reaction occurs, a third concentration, higher than the other two, is administered. If neither you nor the examiner notes any reactions during the three tests, the food is presumed safe, and the testing continues with another food.

Reactions to foods that cause sensitivities may be similar in the laboratory to the reactions you might experience during your usual day—headaches, irritability, sleepiness, disorientation, or even hallucinations. However, sometimes an entirely different symptom from the usual ones appears during the testing. The severity of your reaction depends on how sensitive you are and on the particular concentration of the food extract used. A definite reaction at any of the three concentrations tested indicates a sensitivity.

If you do discover a sensitivity, the examiner can then search for a neutralizing dose. Using different dilutions of the same food extract, he can determine the proper concentration to relieve your symptoms.

Usually only a few foods can be tested at a time during the sublingual procedure. In fact, if a patient has a strong reaction to a food, it is sometimes better to stop the testing and continue it on another day, both to improve the accuracy of the test and to prevent putting too much stress on the body.

A variation of the sublingual test can be used to check your sensitivity to some chemicals and inhalants. It involves your sniffing small amounts of whatever substance you are testing and waiting ten minutes for a response.

One of the foremost advocates of sublingual testing in the United States is Dr. Marshall Mandell of Norwalk, Connecticut.

The following case histories, which he has reported on in medical literature, show how sublingual testing works.

THE CHOCAHOLIC

While treating eight-year-old Allan for an allergy to insect stings, Dr. Mandell learned that the child was lethargic, uninterested in school, and a daydreamer. In addition, he suffered from itching eyes and a dry cough early in the day.

When Allan's mother discussed his diet, it became apparent to Dr. Mandell that food might be playing a role in some of these symptoms. For breakfast Allan would eat a cold oat cereal every day—usually two bowls full—and dry handfuls of it at other times. At lunch he would start with chocolate milk, move on to chocolate ice cream, and finish with chocolate chip cookies. Dr. Mandell decided to do sublingual testing. The first test involved chocolate, which had been removed from Allan's diet five days before the test. Less than an hour after eating it, Allan became tired and confused and developed hives. On a later visit Dr. Mandell tested an oat extract; it produced the itching eyes and the coughing that had plagued Allan often in the morning.

Eliminating these offending foods freed Allan of the symptoms.

A MEAN WITCH

A second patient, a thirty-one-year-old nursery schoolteacher named R.B. who suffered from fatigue, irritability and chronic nasal symptoms, among other things, came to see Dr. Mandell. Her sublingual tests were conclusive and convincing. Egg extract made her so tense that she described herself as a "mean witch"; rice caused everything from chills to generalized abdominal cramps; wheat and chocolate made her feel nauseated and chilly, gave her headaches and clammy hands, and left her so confused that she could no longer spell simple words correctly; and corn caused headaches, chills, moist hands and belching.

As a result of these tests, Dr. Mandell hospitalized R.B. and supervised a fast for eleven days. After the fast he placed her on a rotation diet (see pages 106–109), and she soon was free of symptoms.

Characteristics of Sublingual Testing

ADVANTAGES

1. Sublingual testing reproduces the symptoms of the actual sensitivity. The indirect signs of sensitivity established by pulse testing or kinesiologic testing are generally not as convincing as the direct, recognizable effects obtained by sublingual testing. The procedure of putting a drop of food extract into the mouth; eliciting a response in the form, perhaps, of a splitting headache; and turning it off with the neutralizing dose is as strong an indication of sensitivity as it is possible to receive.

2. The test's ability to determine a neutralizing dose may be useful in the treatment of sensitivities.

3. Sublingual testing is carried out in relatively stable surroundings; this narrows the variables in the testing and increases the accuracy of the test.

4. Technicians are used who are skilled in interpreting reactions to various substances.

5. A variation of sublingual testing—the sniff test—can be used to determine sensitivities to certain chemicals.

DISADVANTAGES

1. Because sublingual testing usually requires at least thirty minutes for each food—and possibly more if a reaction occurs—it is time-consuming. It may take days, sometimes weeks, to test every food under consideration (particularly if many strong reactions occur).

2. As with the intradermal provocative test, sublingual testing is relatively expensive because of the time, personnel and equipment involved.

3. If you are being tested for an assumed problem which forces you to spend several hours a day for a number of days in an unfamiliar laboratory setting, sooner or later you may get restless and fidgety. You may get headaches and may react poorly to the clinical nature of the testing. As a result, even though many

external factors which intensify your symptoms at home are removed by your laboratory stay, new ones may arise to ruin the accuracy of the testing. However, these symptoms can be distinguished from symptoms caused by sensitivities in that the latter will respond to a neutralizing dose.

4. Since food extracts are being used, the test can determine sensitivities only to those portions of a food that can be dissolved.

Cytotoxic Testing

In the cytotoxic test, live white blood cells are mixed with a food extract. The white blood cells react if the extract is from an offending food, but remain normal if the food is safe.

Devised by Dr. A. P. Black and modified by Dr. William Bryan in the late 1950s, cytotoxic testing is based on the observation that living white blood cells can be damaged or destroyed when brought into contact with foods to which one is sensitive.

When a foreign substance (called an antigen) enters the bloodstream, certain white blood cells may produce specific proteins (called antibodies) which can neutralize the antigen and prevent it from harming the body. This antigen-antibody reaction is the basis for vaccines such as the polio vaccine, in which inactivated polio viruses (antigens) are ingested so that the body can form antibodies against them. Should you be exposed to live polio viruses later on, your body can immediately produce antibodies to neutralize the viruses, as a result of its previous exposure to the vaccine.

The antigen-antibody reaction is designed to protect the body, but it can sometimes go awry. In cases of hay fever, for example, the antibodies react with pollen (an antigen), even though pollen is usually not harmful. Symptoms such as a runny nose, watery, itching eyes, and sneezing can result from this interaction.

Similarly, if you are sensitive to a particular food, you may have formed antibodies against it. The struggle between your antibodies and the food (antigen) may set up a series of chemical reactions that damage or destroy some of your white blood cells.

The cytotoxic test measures this reaction. (However, not all food sensitivities are linked to antigen-antibody reactions, and these will not be detected by cytotoxic testing.)

THE TEST

Prior to the cytotoxic test, you must avoid eating for at least twelve hours before a blood sample is drawn. (You may drink minimal amounts of water, if necessary.) In consultation with the physician or his technician, you determine which foods will be tested from a list of available food extracts. The technician will usually select the obvious candidates—such as corn, wheat, milk, egg and beef. From the rest of the foods on the list you simply mark the ones you eat habitually—at least once a week.

As you make your selection of foods to be tested, remember that certain food substances are present in many products; you could be eating them without knowing it. These substances— such as baker's yeast (used in the baking of almost all breads and cakes) and brewer's yeast (an ingredient of many nutritional supplements)—should also be tested.

After the technician has drawn the blood sample, he separates the white blood cells and the plasma, which contains the antibodies, from the rest of the blood. He then places a drop of this mixture on previously prepared slides containing dried extracts of the foods you have selected. (He has also prepared a separate slide of white blood cells alone to compare with the slides containing foods.) When these slides are examined under a microscope, the changes caused by any sensitivity become clear. Slides which contain concentrates of foods to which you are not sensitive remain unchanged; those which contain foods to which you are sensitive may show a variety of reactions, some of which indicate deterioration of the white blood cells.

The destruction of white blood cells as witnessed on the slides is seldom an all-or-nothing phenomenon. In fact, the technician can actually gauge the degree of sensitivity by the number of white blood cells that have been affected. Sensitivities are rated 0 to 4, as follows:

0—*no reaction.* The cells on the slide with the food are the same as those on the slide of white blood cells alone, which means that you are not sensitive to the food.

1—*borderline reaction.* Few of the cells on the slide have been affected, indicating a minimal degree of sensitivity.

2—*slight reaction.* Approximately one-third of the white blood cells are affected, indicating a mild degree of sensitivity.

3—*moderate reaction.* About one-half of the white blood cells are affected, indicating a moderate degree of sensitivity.

4—*marked reaction.* The majority of the cells are affected, indicating a severe degree of sensitivity.

We ourselves have used the cytotoxic food test for hundreds of patients. Let's look at two of our cases that illustrate how cytotoxic testing works.

HE COULDN'T BELIEVE THE DIFFERENCE

Mrs. G, an attractive twenty-nine-year-old woman, functioned quite well despite a host of physical and psychological problems that had dogged her for ten years. Finally she decided to do something about them. For her psychological problems she began to visit a psychotherapist, who attempted to deal with her bouts of depression, nervous exhaustion, fits of crying, and general lack of energy and ambition. For her rashes, stuffy nose and eczema she went to an allergist, who began to treat her for allergies to pollens, dust and molds.

Still Mrs. G remained depressed and anxious; neither did her skin problems improve. Finally someone recommended that she come to us.

When Mrs. G visited our offices, we observed that both her general physical health and her description of her symptoms pointed to brain sensitivities. Indeed, Mrs. G was smoking one and a half packs of cigarettes a day. She craved rich, creamy foods, ice cream, dark breads, cereals, skim milk, and some green vegetables. She was taking Valium daily to alleviate her anxiety.

We drew Mrs. G's blood and ran a cytotoxic test. We were not surprised when the test showed multiple strong sensitivities. She was sensitive to wheat, milk, cashew nuts, honey, yogurt, baker's yeast, mushrooms and cucumbers. Mrs. G's sensitivities were clearly affecting her health. We suggested she stop eating those foods to which she was sensitive and that she stop—or at least cut down on—smoking. In addition, we prescribed a regular regimen of vitamins and minerals.

Within two months Mrs. G had undergone a drastic change, one so complete that her husband called to tell us that he couldn't believe the difference in her condition. She had stuck to our diet, had cut down to three cigarettes per day, and had taken the suggested nutritional supplements. In spite of the fact that she had stopped going to the psychotherapist and the allergist and no longer took Valium, her depression and anxiety had disappeared, her skin problems were gone, and she had found a new zest for life.

THE PRICE OF MR. J'S SUCCESS

Another dramatic case was that of Mr. J, who was on the verge of dropping out of law school when he came to see us. The problem was not his academic work, which was quite good, but the price he seemed to be paying for this success: frequently recurring migraine and tension headaches. The migraines struck with a force that literally disabled him for upwards of twenty-four hours, during which he could do nothing but lie quietly in a darkened room. The tension headaches, which gripped his temples like a vise, were agonizing, though not so devastating.

Mr. J had suffered from these headaches for many years, and he was certain that stress played a key role in triggering his pain. Although he had obtained some relief with medication, neither the pills he took nor the many specialists he consulted seemed to be able to eliminate the headaches.

He had long wanted to be a lawyer and had endured the many headaches in college in order to get this far, but the first six months of law school had taken him to the limits of his tolerance for pain. The idea of continuing in this state for two and a half more years was too much for him.

Cytotoxic testing, which was done the day after his initial consultation with us, showed that Mr. J was highly sensitive to corn; moderately sensitive to honey, wheat and Swiss cheese; mildly sensitive to cucumbers and coffee; and minimally sensitive to lettuce and coconut.

On our advice he eliminated these foods completely. At the end of one week he had already noticed a difference—fewer and definitely less severe headaches. This trend continued, and by the third week he was practically free of headaches. He was able from that point on to continue his law studies without the agony and incapacity he had previously suffered. On the rare occasions when he did get headaches, they were more easily managed.

Characteristics of Cytotoxic Testing

ADVANTAGES

1. Cytotoxic testing demands a minimal investment of time and effort on the part of the patient. (Compare the few moments needed to extract a sample of blood to, for example, the time required for a complete series of sublingual tests.) This is particularly important in the cases of psychotic patients or in hyperactive children, where obtaining lengthy, consistent cooperation is a problem.

2. The test is efficient. One technician can examine between 150 and 250 food tests every day, and patients can receive results on the same day the test is administered.

3. The test is perfectly safe. The potentially toxic foods are added to separated blood, rather than given directly to the patient, as in most other types of sensitivity tests.

4. The observed reactions are relatively objective. No subjective responses from the patient are needed to complete the test.

5. Testing can be repeated, if necessary, with little hardship for the patient.

6. The test picks up some latent food sensitivities that are sometimes missed by other types of tests. This means that certain foods which may cause symptoms only under specific circumstances may appear as sensitivities on the cytotoxic test.

7. For some patients the results of an objective test carry more weight and credibility than those of the more subjective tests.

8. The test can be used for some chemicals, as well as for foods.

DISADVANTAGES

1. Cytotoxic testing does not reproduce symptoms in the way that deliberate food testing and sublingual testing do; thus it is sometimes harder to convince patients of the relationship between certain foods and their symptoms and to get them to comply unreservedly with therapeutic measures.

2. In some diagnostic tests for brain sensitivity the potential treatment is intrinsic in the diagnostic procedure. Fasting, for example, will actually rid most people of their symptoms before they even discover the causes; and sublingual or intradermal provocative testing can establish a neutralizing dose which can prevent or treat symptoms that develop in response to future exposures to the food. Cytotoxic testing, on the other hand, has no element of treatment.

3. The test may give false negative readings for foods to which a patient is clearly sensitive, but which he has not eaten for several months. The apparent reason for this is that antibodies to a particular food begin to disappear during a period when there is no exposure; then, when exposure recurs, the antibodies may return within one or two feedings, and the symptoms will begin again.

4. The test requires a laboratory facility. Because the blood sample must be fresh, you cannot send it by mail; you must appear in person at one of the specialized laboratories.

5. Although the test is less expensive than some of the others, it is more expensive than the home methods of diagnosis.

6. Food sensitivities which cause reactions that are not linked to antigen-antibody reactions will not be picked up by the cytotoxic test.

7. Since only the soluble portion of a food is found in the food extract, reactions to insoluble portions will not be picked up.

The Radio-Allergo-Sorbant Test (RAST)

One of the reasons for the refusal of traditional allergists to accept the notion of the widespread presence of food sensitivities has been medicine's inability to discover antibodies for the offending foods. However, some recent discoveries have begun to change this situation.

The radio-allergo-sorbant test—or RAST—has only recently been applied to the investigation of food sensitivities. Developed in the late 1960s, the RAST measures the number of antibodies the blood contains to specific foods or other allergens.

A number of different kinds of proteins exist in the bloodstream, each with a different function. The proteins involved in defensive functions (the antibodies) are called gamma globulins or immunoglobulins. At present, five classes of immunoglobulins are recognized, each with different chemical and functional characteristics. One of these, an antibody called *IgE* which was discovered in 1966, comprises only about 0.05 percent of all the immunoglobulins. Because it exists in such small quantities, IgE couldn't even be located and identified until new and sophisticated methods of detection became available.

IgE seems to work by attacking the antigens responsible for hay fever and other allergic reactions. In addition, IgE molecules often react with specific food antigens in certain individuals. It is this reaction that the highly sensitive RAST picks up.

The RAST works by a technique which labels the antigen-antibody reaction with a radioactive substance. The intensity of the reaction can then be measured by a Geiger-counter–like device.

At present, RAST materials for only a limited number of foods are available in the United States. Furthermore, the presence of IgE antibodies does not always coincide with clinical symptoms. Nevertheless, the RAST does offer a new and promising approach to the problem of food sensitivities, and it may help to bridge the gap between clinical ecologists and clinical immunologists. The advantages and disadvantages of the RAST are similar to those of cytotoxic testing.

	Fasting and Deliberate Food Testing	Elimination Testing	Pulse Test	Kinesiologic Test	Intradermal Provocative Testing	Sublingual Testing	Cytotoxic Testing / RAST Testing
Eliminates symptoms	✓	✓					
Is capable of reproducing symptoms	✓	✓			✓	✓	
Detoxifies	✓						
Includes component of treatment	✓	✓			✓	✓	
Immediate results				✓			✓
Performed quickly				✓			✓
No expense involved	✓	✓	✓	✓			
Can be used for chemicals and inhalants			✓	✓	✓	✓	✓
Objective			✓	✓	✓		✓
Can be performed at home	✓	✓	✓	✓			
Helps to uncover hidden or masked sensitivities	✓	✓	✓	✓	✓	✓	✓
Relatively unaffected by environmental conditions					✓		✓

DISADVANTAGES

	Fasting and Deliberate Food Testing	Elimination Testing	Pulse Test	Kinesiologic Test	Intradermal Provocative Testing	Sublingual Testing	Cytotoxic Testing / RAST Testing
Withdrawal	✓	✓	✓				
Detoxification symptoms	✓						
Does not reproduce symptoms			✓	✓			✓
No component of treatment			✓	✓			✓
Delayed results	✓	✓	✓		✓	✓	
Test is lengthy	✓	✓	✓		✓	✓	
Not safe for everyone	✓	✓			✓	✓	
Expense involved					✓	✓	✓
Generally cannot be used for chemicals and inhalants	✓	✓					
Subjective	✓	✓		✓	✓	✓	
Cannot be performed at home					✓	✓	✓
Requires enemas	✓						
Can miss delayed sensitivities	✓	✓	✓	✓	✓	✓	✓
Uses water-soluble form of food					✓	✓	✓
Influenced by external conditions	✓	✓	✓	✓		✓	
Must stop smoking	✓	✓	✓				

SEVEN:
Complications

In many instances diagnosing brain sensitivity is as simple as it sounds. Many people are sensitive to just one or two easily detectable substances, and their symptoms can be relieved simply by avoiding contact with those substances.

But, as we have implied, there are other cases of sensitivity that are not so easy to identify. Sometimes sensitivities mask each other; sometimes a person is sensitive to something so obscure and esoteric that finding it requires a major search into his personal history and life-style; and sometimes symptoms that seem at first to be caused by sensitivities turn out to be primarily psychological in nature. In addition, there are times when a test can accurately pinpoint a sensitivity to a specific food, but if you later decide to check out your results by eating that food, you may experience no adverse reactions. This may tempt you to disregard the results of the test, not realizing that some reactions can be delayed or blocked in various ways.

Such problems can interfere with both your testing and your interpretation of the results. Therefore, let's examine some of the complications that might impede your search for sensitivities.

Combination Sensitivities

As we have noted, there are times when a specific sensitivity reaction such as a headache is caused by a combination of different foods rather than by a single food. A brain sensitivity is not a fixed entity. Before it can produce symptoms, it has to reach a certain threshold. It's as if there is a point system in which each food to which you are sensitive has a numerical value. The more severe the sensitivity, the higher the value. Before you actually suffer the symptoms of, say, a headache, you have to accumulate a certain number of points.

How would this work? Let's assume that you need 10 points to experience the symptoms of a headache. You are sensitive to the following foods, with the following hypothetical point values: tomato—12; apple—10; milk—7; orange—7; raisins—5; cucumbers—4; coffee—3. Tests such as kinesiology may indicate that you are sensitive to all these foods. But, because of your threshold of 10, only tomatoes or apples are strong enough to precipitate a headache when they are eaten alone. Neither milk nor the other four foods, on the other hand, would cause a headache unless they were eaten in combinations that would add up to 10 points or more.

The point system applies to chemicals and inhalants as well, so that the situation becomes even more complex if you are also sensitive to auto exhaust (5) and ragweed (3). Any combination of foods, chemicals and inhalants adding up to 10 or more points can produce the symptoms; any combination adding up to fewer than 10 will leave you symptom-free. For example, hay fever sufferers who have eliminated their food allergens may notice a decline or disappearance of their hay fever even during the height of the pollen season because their total points are below the threshold.

While the point system is hypothetical, its purpose is clear. If a test shows that you are sensitive to milk even though you don't develop symptoms when you drink it, that doesn't necessarily mean that the test is unreliable; it may mean that milk will only give you symptoms in the appropriate combination with other substances to which you are sensitive. Understanding the point system can help you to more accurately assess your test results.

Stress and Sensitivity Thresholds

Thresholds are not stable; they may increase or decrease, depending on internal and external factors. If your threshold is 10 one day, that doesn't necessarily mean that 10 is a fixed number at which your threshold will always remain.

Many factors can shift the threshold either up or down. One of the most important is the presence or absence of stress. As we noted in the case of Gladys (see pages 12–14), when we have the capacity to resist the negative effects of stress, our thresholds are raised; however, when stress takes its toll on us, it can push our threshold down.

Much of the problem of brain sensitivity actually revolves around our ability to adapt to and overcome stress. This constant process of meeting and reacting to threats to our well-being was described by Dr. Hans Selye in his pioneering work *The Stress of Life.* Dr. Selye described stress as not only the psychological problems we usually think of—those "stressful situations" that cause nervous tension—but as wear and tear of all kinds during the normal process of living (such as exposure to heat and cold, infections, pain, exposure to toxins, work responsibilities, pressures from family and friends, and the aging process itself). A certain amount of stress is normal and even beneficial. But excessive and constant stress can exhaust our bodies' defenses, leaving us open to the physical and psychological symptoms of brain sensitivity.

Selye described the three stages we may go through in response to *stress, alarm, adaptation,* and *exhaustion.* During the alarm phase, we first confront something potentially harmful to our lives. Our body reacts to the danger by releasing hormones, such as adrenalin (from the adrenal glands), into our system in an effort to deal with the situation. Then, as the body begins to stabilize, the second phase, adaptation, sets in. The adrenal glands—the glands of stress—now secrete cortisone-like hormones. During this phase we have successfully adapted to the source of the stress, and our bodies continue to do whatever is necessary to keep us on an even keel. Normally, we can confine most stresses to this second, adaptive phase. We react, control, and maintain stability for as long as the stress exists. But what happens if the stress persists or is too overwhelming for our bodies to manage? What happens if the stress is bolstered and strengthened by other stresses, and the combination grows too strong for us to handle? At that point, we enter the third phase of reaction to stress: exhaustion (inability of the adrenal glands to continue normal functioning).

Exhaustion is the phase in which the threshold is lowered and the foods to which we are sensitive (themselves stressors) become simply straws breaking the camel's back. The sensitivity/stress relationship can turn into a powerful, vicious cycle: something lowers our resistance; combined stresses inhibit our capacity to adapt; we become susceptible to new stresses—like brain sensitivities—that we might otherwise be able to handle; and the new stresses lower our defenses still further, rendering us susceptible to serious illness.

The character and the amount of stress in your life, then, are elements that can affect the results of your testing. Other factors that similarly affect the threshold include the biorhythmic cycles, the menstrual cycle, and the general state of your health and nutrition.

At times it is possible to raise your threshold by ingesting certain vitamins, such as vitamin C and vitamin B-6, before you eat an offending food. While the vitamins' blocking action can prove beneficial in the long run (see pages 110–111), it can also work against you while you are testing. If, for example, just before you test something to which you are sensitive, you eat a food rich in vitamin C, the vitamin may prevent you from reacting, either by blocking the reaction completely or by lowering the "point value" of the food so that the reaction cannot take place. The absence of a reaction might lead you to believe mistakenly that something is safe for you when actually it is not. It is therefore a good idea to retest any suspected food that turns out negative on the initial testing.

Chemical Interference

The piece of orange that causes you to feel lethargic or mildly depressed may not be the simple, innocuous citrus fruit you thought it was; instead, it may have been injected with a dye to give the skin more eye appeal. Dye injected into living fruit does more than settle into the skins; it pushes on into the meat of the fruit itself. Therefore, your sensitivity might not be to the orange at all, but to the artificial cosmetic additive.

As we have mentioned before, additives such as the dye in oranges; preservatives such as BHA and BHT in cereals and other grain products; flavor enhancers such as MSG; artificial flavors; artificial colors; artificial odor producers, such as the ones that produce the oven-fresh smell of some commercial breads; and a whole range of other chemicals and mixtures that are found in the foods we eat are capable of producing sensitivity reactions. Literally thousands of these chemicals are added to foods by the commercial food industry.

In addition, preservatives such as BHA or BHT may be added to the packaging material rather than to the foods. Although this allows the manufacturer to delete BHA, BHT, etc., from the list of ingredients, a significant percentage of the preservative does nevertheless enter the food.

Many potentially harmful substances routinely find their way unintentionally into our food. For example, pesticides that are sprayed over apple crops to protect them from insect infestation are transferred from the orchard to our bodies by means of the innocent apple. As we all know, these additives can be quite harmful. Some are suspected of causing cancer and other serious diseases, and some are implicated in both mild and severe brain sensitivities. The case history of Mrs. D (see pages 47–48) is a good example. Mrs. D, who gave up meat in order to stay awake during the evening, was aware that cattle are often injected with hormones or are fed chemicals to increase their weight, and she wondered whether she was sensitive to the meat itself or to something that had been added to it. Shortly after we discovered her meat sensitivity, she managed to find some meat that had come from organically raised steers and found that she could eat it without any ill effects. Unfortunately she couldn't get the unadulterated meat on a regular basis, so she decided to remain a vegetarian.

When you begin to test foods, make sure you test them in the same state in which you usually eat them. If you generally eat nonorganic foods that contain additives, those are the foods you should test. If, however, you find you are sensitive to one of these foods, run a second test on the same food that has been organically grown to determine whether your sensitivity is due to the food itself or to chemical additives in the food.

Food additives are only one of the ways in which chemicals can interfere with your testing. Just as we are unaware of all the additives in our food, most of us do not realize the extent to which we are surrounded by chemicals. Not only are they present in lipstick, after-shave lotion, shampoos, deodorants, and various cleaning products—and as fillers in many tablets (vitamins as well as medications)—they are also an integral part of synthetic rugs, furnishings and clothing. It is possible to become sensitive to any one—or any combination—of these chemicals.

If you are testing yourself, it is easy to overlook everyday items that may contain chemicals. Wool draperies, for instance, when sent to the cleaners are often sprayed with a moth preventative. Your clothing as well may not only be woven from synthetic material (dacron, nylon, various plastics) to which you have developed a sensitivity, but may have been treated with chemicals before being sold—chemicals that are not mentioned on the label. A process for making permanent press clothing calls for the items to be soaked in formaldehyde, creased in the appropriate places, and then baked in ovens. The baking gets rid of most of the formaldehyde, but not all. Some people may break out in rashes when they come in contact with permanent press clothing;

others may suffer from brain sensitivities. For these reasons it is a good idea to wash new clothes before you wear them.

Finally, chemicals can interfere with accurate test results when someone is either unwilling or unable to remove a sensitizing chemical from his environment during the testing. This next case history makes the point.

YES, WE HAVE NO CIGARETTES

Mr. E was eager to find help for his thirty-year-old daughter Lisa, who had been in and out of psychiatric hospitals for ten years. Lisa herself felt that she was beyond help. At the time of her first psychotic breakdown when she was twenty years old, she had been diagnosed as a paranoid schizophrenic. In her more lucid moments she described her life as miserable and complained bitterly about the voices which, for ten years, had not left her alone. The voices were both male and female; they kept up a constant barrage of verbal abuse—all directed at her. For example, if she went to the bathroom, they would torment her from the toilet paper. If she tried to cook, they would assail her from the pots and pans. Often they urged her to kill herself, and her frequent periods of hospitalization were generally preceded by some self-destructive act.

Lisa was also extremely hyperactive, not being able to sit still for more than a few minutes at a time. During her ten-year history, doctors had tried many methods of treatment, including electric shock therapy, drug therapy, and behavior modification therapy; but none had had any influence on her bizarre behavior or auditory hallucinations. Finally Mr. E brought Lisa to see us.

Our testing revealed a number of problems, including a low blood sugar condition (hypoglycemia). As part of our treatment for hypoglycemia, we advise that our patients avoid sugar, caffeine, alcohol and nicotine. Lisa consumed large quantities of sugar and caffeine, drank moderate amounts of wine, and smoked two to three packs of cigarettes a day. Although she agreed, under pressure, to go along with other aspects of the overall treatment plan, she refused to give up any of these four items.

In addition to her hallucinations and hyperactivity, Lisa had skin allergies, insomnia, digestive problems, and circulatory problems. Much to her surprise, these symptoms began to clear up when she followed the part of the treatment plan to which she had agreed. Encouraged, she tried to comply with the rest of the treatment program; after eliminating sugar, caffeine and alcohol from her diet, she noted an even greater sense of well-being. The voices, however, persisted in full fury, as did her restlessness. When we first suggested that there might be a connection between these remaining symptoms and the cigarettes she was smoking, she refused to listen. But finally she agreed to give them up, with the understanding that if she did stop smoking for the two to three weeks we had suggested and noted no relief, she would be allowed to smoke again without interference. We all agreed, and Lisa began to wean herself from cigarettes. When she had gone three weeks without smoking, she returned to our office and announced that the voices were as loud, as vicious, and as persistent as before. Her father confirmed that Lisa had not smoked a single cigarette during those three weeks.

At that point we were prepared to agree that Lisa's remaining symptoms were not related to tobacco, and we would have said so had it not been for her unintentional help. She had brought a pack of cigarettes with her so that she could start smoking again as soon as our session was over. As she began to search through her purse for the cigarettes, we noticed that she had a pipe in her bag. We asked about it, and Mr. E explained that he was a pipe smoker and owned a large pipe collection. Pipe smoking seemed a lot safer to him than cigarette smoking, and, to help Lisa forgo her cigarettes, he had given her one of his pipes and encouraged her to use it instead. For the past three weeks Lisa had been smoking pipefuls of tobacco each day. Neither of them had volunteered this information because they felt it was irrelevant, and we didn't ask about it because it didn't occur to us that Lisa might be smoking a pipe.

We explained forcefully that Lisa had to forgo *all* forms of tobacco so that we could make an accurate evaluation of its effect on her brain. It was no easy matter to convince her, but in the end she acquiesced. Mr. E also agreed not to smoke a pipe when she was with him and to confine all his smoking either to the outdoors or to one room in the house to which she would not have access.

Ten days later we received a phone call from Mr. E. He told us that Lisa was completely free of the voices and that she was no longer hyperactive. A few days later they both returned for a consultation. The transformation in Lisa was extraordinary: the psychotic look was gone from her eyes; she was able to sit calmly; and her compulsive pacing was gone. She spoke clearly and coherently as she reviewed the horror of the past ten years of her life. She could hardly believe that she had so quickly and so definitely emerged from the grip of psychosis and the enslavement of the voices.

Could tobacco really have had such a powerful and dramatic effect? Additional proof came a few months later when Lisa developed a medical problem requiring a short period of hospitalization. In the hospital she was surrounded by people who smoked, and finally she accepted one of the many offers of a cigarette. One cigarette led to another, and within three days the voices and the agitation returned. Although she remembered that she had been free of the voices when she had stopped smoking, Lisa's judgment was impaired by the cigarettes, and it was just as difficult for her to give them up a second time. When she finally succeeded, the voices stopped within a week.

The Fungus Connection

Fungi can also play a role in brain sensitivity. When a food is overgrown with fungus, you can see it—the molds on cheese or bread, for example—but more often fungal growth is so small it cannot be detected by the naked eye. Most of the time your immune system is capable of dealing with the invading organism. But it is also possible to develop a sensitivity to these fungi, even though the food itself, if free of the fungus, would not cause symptoms.

It should be noted that it is also possible for a fungus growing within your own body to become a source of many neurological and emotional symptoms should you develop a brain sensitivity to it. A recent paper in the medical literature reported on a series of such cases. Where such infections exist or are suspected, medical treatment should be sought.

Temporary Loss of Sensitivity

Many (but not all) food sensitivities affecting the brain are of such a nature that they may temporarily lose their ability to produce symptoms if the foods have not been eaten for a period of anywhere from a few weeks to a few months (the time varies from individual to individual and from food to food). Foods that fall into this category may give false negative results during testing.

To avoid being fooled by this complication, remember that getting no reaction to a food which you have not eaten for a few weeks does not necessarily mean the food is safe. Each of these foods should be tested at least twice in a three-day period. (The longer it has been since you last ate the food, the more frequently you should test it.) Assume that the food is safe only if you remain symptom-free after several tests.

Delayed responses of this nature can occur for several reasons. Sometimes foods are harmful only after they have reached a certain concentration in your system. When you first eat such a food after a prolonged period of abstinence, you may not ingest a concentration high enough to cause a reaction; only after eating it over a period of time will your body begin to react.

Another cause of delayed responses has to do with the fact that some foods (such as wheat) may be inefficiently absorbed into the bloodstream from the intestine, and it may take several feedings before the body has consumed enough to react.

Sometimes, too, offending food can damage the lining of the intestine (intestinal mucosa). If the food has not been eaten for a long period, the mucosa may heal. The first time the food is eaten again, it may redamage the intestinal lining, setting up the conditions necessary for brain sensitivity on subsequent eating.

Whatever the reason for this complication, the solution lies in retesting suspicious foods that the initial test indicates may be safe.

Major Versus Minor Sensitivities

Some of the substances to which you are sensitive may cause such strong reactions (major sensitivity) that they overshadow those which elicit relatively mild responses (minor sensitivity). As a result the latter may be missed in testing.

In fact, major brain sensitivities can at times actually cause the brain tissue to ignore the milder sensitizing agents. Thus the minor sensitivities may at first go undetected; they may not surface until the major offending agents have been eliminated.

Built-in Limitations

Each of the tests we have described has its advantages and disadvantages. And none of the tests is absolutely certain to pick up all sensitivities. Fasting and deliberate food testing, for example, cannot uncover chemical or inhalant sensitivities (unless the chemicals are in the foods), while the cytotoxic and RAST tests, which measure the reactions of white blood cells and antibodies, can only detect sensitivities that affect these systems. Occasionally you might have to try more than one type of test to be sure you have a complete picture of the nature and extent of your sensitivities. See the chart at the end of Chapter Six for a summary of the advantages and disadvantages of each of the tests.

Mind Over Matter

Although it is a potent factor in much of what we term illness, brain sensitivity is by no means responsible for all mental symptoms. Some people find it difficult to accept the fact that their problems are indeed rooted in their emotions and eagerly seek physical explanations for all of their suffering. These people may be tempted to continue searching for sensitivities even when none exist. Such efforts not only are unrewarding, but may actually interfere with their search for appropriate help.

Often a combination of physical and emotional factors can lead to the development of symptoms. Being aware of as many of these factors as possible gives you the best chance of making an accurate diagnosis and of beginning the most effective program of treatment.

EIGHT:
Treatment

A brain sensitivity may indicate not only that your brain is reacting adversely to one or more substances, but that there may be
some other problem with your body that makes you susceptible
to such a sensitivity in the first place. All too often our efforts at
healing are directed at removing symptoms rather than dealing
with their causes. If you have a painful splinter in your finger, you
know that it is better to remove the splinter than to leave it alone
and take pain killers. Yet we often reach for an aspirin rather than
deal with the stress that causes our tension headache, or swallow
antacids rather than eat more sensibly. Likewise, when it comes
to brain sensitivity, there is a tendency to want to get rid of the
discomfort, lethargy or anxiety without coming to grips with its
basic cause.

There are a number of methods of removing the symptoms of
brain sensitivity without addressing the factors that predispose us
to them. Although we favor the use of these methods, we feel they
are most effective when used in conjunction with a thorough
evaluation and a treatment program that deals with the whole
person. Brain sensitivities do not occur in a vacuum; they can be
influenced by numerous internal and environmental factors. Anything that detracts from your optimum level of health, such as
overwork or infection, can lower your threshold and make you
more susceptible. In addition, certain specific abnormalities, such
as hypothyroidism and nutritional deficiencies, can also encourage

their development. The most fundamental treatment of brain sensitivities involves correcting these underlying abnormalities.

Specifically, how can we treat sensitivities? Let's assume that you have a sensitivity to wheat which produces the symptom of anxiety. The sensitivity can be treated on three basic levels:

1. *Removal of the symptom*—for example, taking a tranquilizer to overcome anxiety. Because this approach treats only the symptom and ignores the possible relationship between wheat and anxiety, the other detrimental effects of eating wheat—many of which may be hidden for the time being—go uncorrected.

2. *Recognition of the relationship between the symptom and the offending agent*—by removing or preventing the negative effects of wheat through one of four methods: elimination, rotation dieting, neutralization or blocking. These methods may remove the anxiety and any other symptoms caused by wheat, but they do not necessarily change the factors that led to a sensitivity to wheat in the first place. Nevertheless, they are far superior to the symptom-removal method.

3. *Treating the factors that cause the sensitivity*—an approach that not only removes the overt and hidden symptoms but aims at freeing us from the sensitivity itself. In so doing, it improves our overall health as well. Unfortunately, with our present level of knowledge, we cannot always effect treatment at this level.

As a rule, we do not favor the first approach, particularly if it is used by itself. We prefer the second and third, sometimes individually, but more often in combination. Both approaches have their own strengths and limitations.

Direct Treatment of Sensitivity Reactions

ELIMINATION DIETS

Eliminating the offending agent (food, chemical or inhalant) is the most obvious way of dealing with a brain sensitivity.

Elimination works well in many cases. However, it is not always the most appropriate or most effective treatment when used by itself. Certainly if gas fumes from your stove are causing symptoms, it may be necessary to replace the gas range with an electric one. Similarly, if celery is the only thing you have found that gives you headaches, eliminating celery may be the most reasonable course of action. But what happens if you have discovered sensitivities to wheat, corn and milk? Eliminating these three basic foods from your diet would place enormous restrictions on what you could eat. And many people are sensitive to a number of other foods as well—to fifteen, twenty, or even more. The restrictions caused by eliminating them all could become a heavy burden. Some people feel that if getting rid of their symptoms means going through that kind of bother, the treatment isn't worth the cure.

There is, however, an alternative to indefinitely eliminating offending foods: a rotation diet, which, after a period of initial abstinence, permits you to eat them on a regular, though controlled, basis.

ROTATION DIETS

In contrast to a few days of fasting, which leaves your body even more susceptible to offending foods, a prolonged period of abstinence (weeks or months) can prevent the appearance of symptoms when you next eat the offending food. In fact, it may take several feedings over the next few days before your symptoms recur. Once they do reappear, however, they are likely to remain, or to recur each time you eat that food, even if you allow a few days between feedings. At that point it would take a second period of prolonged abstinence before you could again eat the food without suffering symptoms.

If you go through a period of abstinence that leaves you free of symptoms, you can usually continue to eat a particular food if you eat it no more often than once every five days. Although there are some brain sensitivities that do not follow this pattern, the majority do.

It usually takes about four days for traces of whatever food you eat to leave your body; therefore, if you are sensitive to milk and you abstain for a few months and then begin to drink it at least once every two or three days, your body will experience a gradual buildup in the concentration of milk and your symptoms will return. But if you drink milk on Day 1, avoid it for Days 2, 3 and 4 (giving your body time to eliminate it), and drink it again on Day 5, the concentration of milk in your body may remain low enough to avoid causing a reaction.

Most people who benefit from a rotation diet do well on a four-day rotation (allowing three days between eatings of a food). However, people with more severe cases of sensitivity often need a seven-day rotation (six days between eatings). In either case the basic principles necessary for setting up a rotation diet are the same.

To launch a rotation diet, begin by making separate lists of foods for each day of the rotation. First draw a chart of either four or seven columns—depending on whether you are planning a four-day or a seven-day rotation. Next, divide the food families among the columns.

Food families are foods that share certain common characteristics. A person sensitive to one member of the family is often sensitive to other members—this is called a cross-sensitivity. The parsley family, for example, includes carrots, celery, parsnips, dill, caraway and parsley. If you do have a cross-sensitivity, eating carrots on one day of your rotation, celery on a second, parsley on a third, and so on can undermine the therapeutic value of the diet. (See Appendix 2 for a list of these families.)

Cross-sensitivities do not occur in everyone. You can find out if you have a cross-sensitivity by examining the pattern of your known sensitivities to see if they follow family lines. If you do not, you can set up a rotation diet without regard to food families. But if you have any doubts, it is better to take the extra precaution of rotating your foods in family groups.

Finally, apportion all the foods you normally eat or plan to eat among the columns, leaving out the ones to which you are sensitive. (See Appendix 2 for a sample rotation diet.)

Each day, limit your choice of foods to those on the list for that day, as if you were choosing from a menu in a restaurant. You don't have to eat all the foods on that list, but you must limit yourself to only those foods listed. Most people can tolerate eating the same food more than once on a given day. But people who become sensitive particularly rapidly may have to limit themselves to eating each food only once on the day that food is allowed. After several weeks or months, begin to add the offending foods slowly on a rotation basis, making sure that their addition does not cause a recurrence of symptoms.

The exact length of time a food must be eliminated varies considerably, both from individual to individual and from food to food. In most cases six to twelve weeks is enough, although there are some occasions when two weeks is sufficient and others when a year is not enough. The only way you can find out is through trial and error—by periodically retesting the food. When you no longer show a reaction to a particular food, it can be added to your rotation diet.

It may seem simpler to rotate only those foods and food families to which you are sensitive and eat the other foods at will. The problem with this approach is that if you have multiple food sensitivities, you probably have a tendency to develop sensitivities to foods you eat often. As a result, if you rotate only those foods to which you are sensitive and eat other foods on a more frequent basis, you may soon develop new sensitivities to some of the nonrotated foods.

Let's assume, for example, that you have tested yourself and found a sensitivity to wheat and wheat products. You avoid wheat in all forms, and your symptoms disappear. But one or two months later your symptoms come back. When you test yourself again, you find that while your sensitivity to wheat has disappeared, you are now sensitive to corn—a food you are now eating frequently. Eliminating wheat hasn't changed your susceptibility to developing sensitivities; instead, it has caused your body to find another food or chemical to which to react. This problem can be avoided by rotating all of your foods.

Elimination and rotation diets are often effective methods of controlling symptoms of brain sensitivity, but they may not touch the core of the problem. Symptoms produced by foods are often just the tip of the sensitivity iceberg—the visible part of a problem that has hidden, more fundamental ramifications. There are, however, two other ways to overcome sensitivities: You can block or neutralize their effects, or you can pinpoint and correct the underlying problems that caused the sensitivities in the first place. Using one or both of these approaches in conjunction with an elimination or rotation diet often yields positive results when either approach by itself does not.

NEUTRALIZING REACTIONS

As we have noted (Chapter Six, pp. 76–78), the neutralizing dose, which can be determined by sublingual and intradermal provocative testing, is the exact concentration of a sensitizing agent that actually blocks your symptoms.

The neutralizing dose can be used to stop a sensitivity reaction once it has started, but it is more commonly used prophylactically —that is, to prevent the onset of a reaction. If you are sensitive to a number of different substances, a neutralizing dose can be developed for each. The doses can then be mixed together and administered either by injections (which are generally given once or twice a week) or by mouth (by placing a prescribed number of drops under your tongue several times a day).

The long-term therapeutic use of neutralizing doses appears to produce no ill effects. In fact, clinical evidence indicates that continuous use of the neutralizing dose for up to six months or more often seems to increase the body's resistance to the offending foods, chemicals, or inhalants to the point where the neutralizing dose can be discontinued without a return of symptoms.

Administration of the neutralizing dose, however, requires a laboratory (to determine specific concentrations and to prepare adequate amounts for daily use), and there are other ways of blocking sensitizing reactions that do not involve such elaborate procedures.

BLOCKING REACTIONS

Clinical experience has shown that it is often possible to block a sensitivity reaction by using certain specific agents. As with the neutralizing dose, these blocking agents can often stop or greatly diminish a sensitivity reaction. They can even prevent reactions from occurring.

Vitamins C and B-6   We have often been able to block a sensitivity reaction by administering vitamins C and B-6. These vitamins can be given by injection or taken orally. When injected intravenously, they can have an almost instantaneous effect. They can be equally effective when taken orally, but the results take more time.

If we see a patient while he is in the midst of an attack, we sometimes inject the vitamins at a slow, steady pace—particularly if the attack is severe. Often the symptoms disappear while the vitamins are still being injected. In that case we stop the injection no matter how much is left in the syringe, since there is a delicate balance involved in blocking a sensitivity reaction: too little or too much of the blocking agent will not be as effective as the right amount. If the intravenous vitamins are going to work, they usually do so within five to ten minutes of the injection.

When vitamins are taken by mouth to prevent a reaction, they need to be eaten far enough in advance of the food (usually one to one and a half hours) so that they have a chance to be absorbed and ready for action when the food strikes. Similarly, a delay of one to one and a half hours can be expected before the vitamins will stop a brain sensitivity reaction that has already begun. Dosages range from 500 to 3,000 milligrams of vitamin C and from 100 to 3,000 milligrams of vitamin B-6. However, the ingestion of high doses of vitamins may lead to side effects (for example, diarrhea and abdominal cramps with vitamin C), and should be done with caution and under medical supervision.

Mr. K is a friend of ours who discovered through fasting and deliberate food testing that his chronic low-grade depression and sense of fatigue were brought on by eating fish or meat. He liked these foods and furthermore insisted that the business lunches he frequently had to attend made it impractical for him to eliminate them. He was delighted to find that a gram of vitamin C and half a gram of vitamin B-6 taken about one hour before eating these foods completely eliminated their negative effects.

We have noted that in many cases chewing or sucking these vitamins can significantly decrease the one- to one-and-a-half-hour lag time. A possible explanation for this accelerated effect is that material placed under the tongue is more rapidly absorbed into the body.

Sodium and Potassium Bicarbonate The pH of the body is a measure of the body's acidity or alkalinity. A neutral pH is designated by the number 7; an acid pH is less than 7, and an alkaline pH is above 7. As a general rule, when sensitivity and allergy reactions occur, the pH shifts toward the acidic side. Under these circumstances it is often possible to prevent or stop a brain sensitivity reaction by moving the pH back to a normal level.

A combination of two-thirds sodium bicarbonate (baking soda) and one-third potassium bicarbonate (obtainable at pharmacies) can be used to increase the pH. Where indicated, we recommend that one-fourth to one teaspoon of this mixture be dissolved in a glass of water and taken as soon as possible after an attack has begun. As in the case of oral ingestion of vitamins C and B-6, there is a lag time before the bicarbonate mixture takes effect. Each of these measures should be used only after consultation with a physician.

Neutralizing and blocking approaches can stop most brain sensitivity reactions. However, they are not effective in every case; and even when they work, they do so within certain limitations. The availability of a neutralizing dose or blocking agent for, say, a sensitivity to potatoes does not mean that you have carte blanche to eat potatoes in whatever quantity or frequency you choose, but that you can eat potatoes in moderation. It is still possible to overwhelm the neutralizing or blocking effect by eating too much of an offending food.

Even when neutralizing or blocking approaches work very well on their own, we still encourage people to treat the factors that predispose them to the sensitivity in the first place.

Treating the Predisposing Factors

Just as foods, chemicals and inhalants can adversely affect the brain, causing both psychological and physical symptoms, so ailments of the psyche or body can result in brain sensitivities. Thus, the most effective approach to treating a brain sensitivity is to treat the person as a whole—addressing the body, mind and spirit.

Since an almost endless array of factors can render you susceptible to sensitivities, it is hardly feasible to list them all here. But certain areas are particularly important in predisposing people to brain sensitivities: disorders associated with the digestive and hormonal systems (including hypoglycemia); problems with nutrition (including vitamin and mineral imbalances); lack of exercise; stress; ecological factors; and spiritual influences.

DIGESTIVE DISORDERS

Improper or incomplete digestion is thought to be a prime factor in the development of some cases of brain sensitivity. Clinical evidence supports this view, revealing that many people with food sensitivities also have digestive problems and that when the digestive problems are corrected the food sensitivities disappear. Why this happens is still conjecture. One theory assumes that when food is not digested properly, portions of the partially digested food are absorbed into the bloodstream. There the body recognizes the partially digested material not as food but as a foreign substance, which causes the body's defense mechanism to react. The result is a sensitivity. Another theory has it that foods may contain specific elements which, when they are not broken down as they normally would be during digestion, are capable of provoking a sensitivity response.

Digestive disorders such as these are not limited to the stomach. Problems can occur anywhere along the alimentary canal, from the mouth to the colon.

The Mouth Some people may suffer from brain sensitivities because they don't chew their food properly. They gulp it down in whole, barely masticated pieces. If foods are insufficiently chewed, the saliva, which contains digestive enzymes, does not get a chance to work adequately, increasing the likelihood that partially digested food will be absorbed into the bloodstream.

You can avoid this problem by chewing your food slowly and thoroughly. If solid foods are chewed long enough, they will actually liquefy in the mouth. Liquids should also be given an opportunity to mix with saliva. Thus the adage, "Drink your solid food and chew your liquids."

The Stomach   Any number of gastronomical disorders can have a disruptive effect on digestion. Two common ones relate to levels of acidity and to the stomach's emptying time.

As antacid commercials have been pointing out for decades, an excess of stomach acid—hydrochloric acid—leads to indigestion. But a second lesser known cause of indigestion is the exact opposite—an inadequate amount of hydrochloric acid. A certain amount of hydrochloric acid is actually necessary for proper digestion, and many people, particularly as they get older, are unable to produce enough of it. And even when enough hydrochloric acid is produced, it is not effective unless the food remains in the stomach long enough for the hydrochloric acid to work. If the stomach empties too rapidly, hydrochloric acid simply doesn't have enough time to break the food down.

Each of these conditions can produce food sensitivities, and each can be treated. Excessive acidity can be treated with antacids, while a deficiency of acid (as well as a rapid emptying time) can be treated by swallowing one or more acid tablets (in the form of betaine hydrochloride or glutamic acid) just before eating. Stomach acid tablets, like antacids, are available without prescription at health food stores or pharmacies. But because using antacids for an acid-deficient stomach or acid tablets for an overly acidic stomach can actually exacerbate the problem, neither treatment should be used without proper medical consultation. (Methods for diagnosing these conditions are noted in Appendix 3, pp. 166–168.)

The Pancreas   The pancreas produces a variety of digestive enzymes crucial to adequate digestion in the small intestine. A lack of these enzymes is a prime factor in many cases of brain sensitivity.

In fact, recent findings indicate that a vicious cycle may be set up involving the pancreas and sensitizing agents. Offending foods or chemicals may shock the pancreas into not functioning properly; as a result, digestion is impaired and the sensitivities worsen, which further inhibits the functioning of the pancreas.

To overcome the problem of inadequate production, oral preparations (tablets) of pancreatic enzymes can be taken. The frequency, dose and type of enzymes needed, however, vary from person to person and should be determined by an experienced clinician. Amino acids in the form of capsules, liquid or powder may also be given as supplements to stimulate the production of enzymes.

It is also possible for the production of enzymes to be adequate, but for the enzymes to be inactivated before they have a chance to work because the pH level is not proper. Pancreatic enzymes require an alkaline pH (above 7) to work; they become inactivated by an acid pH (below 7). The small intestine remains alkaline as a result of the sodium and potassium bicarbonate (alkaline materials) the pancreas secretes. If the pancreas is unable to produce enough sodium and potassium bicarbonate, or if too much acid from the stomach enters the small intestine, the pH may be lowered to a point where pancreatic enzymes can lose their effectiveness, even if there are enough of them. This problem can be overcome by drinking a mixture of sodium and potassium bicarbonate (same combination and dosage as mentioned earlier) half an hour after eating.

As with the stomach, pancreatic problems should not be treated without proper medical supervision.

The Colon (Large Intestine)   The colon eliminates wastes from the body, a process vital to life and health. Constipation and other factors that inhibit this process allow toxins to accumulate in the body. These toxins can affect the overall state of your health and leave you more susceptible to sensitizing substances.

In cultures where the diet contains ample amounts of fiber, food is normally eliminated from the body in twenty-four to forty-eight hours. In cultures like our own, where the diet is low in fiber and high in refined carbohydrates, it normally takes forty-eight to ninety-six hours or more for food to leave the body. This prolonged transit time has been associated with constipation, diverticulosis, colon cancer, and other related diseases, as well as with food sensitivities. So it is important that you add enough fiber to your diet (usually in the form of raw fruits and vegetables or whole grains).

Special preparations such as bentonite (available at some health food stores or pharmacies) can also help in detoxification. Bentonite is a type of clay that the Chinese have used for over 1,000 years to remove toxins from the body. When swallowed, it passes through the intestines like a sponge, absorbing toxins many times its own weight, which it then carries out of the body during bowel movements.

The colon is also lined with friendly bacteria that help the body function properly. Antibiotics taken to kill harmful bacteria sometimes also kill the helpful ones. Acidophilus tablets or yogurt which contains live cultures can help restore these bacteria.

HORMONAL DISORDERS

The functions of the body are controlled by two major regulatory systems: the nervous system and the endocrine or hormonal system. Although the systems interrelate, the nervous system is mainly in control of activities that require rapid change (such as the movement of voluntary muscles), while the endocrine system controls the various metabolic functions of the body (such as the chemical reactions in cells).

Because brain sensitivities involve chemical reactions, they are undoubtedly influenced directly by the endocrine system. There is much clinical evidence to indicate that malfunctions of this system are a predisposing factor in the development of brain sensitivities. This is particularly true in relation to the thyroid, thymus, adrenal and gonadal glands.

The Thyroid Gland The thyroid, located in the neck, produces the hormones that control a number of vital functions.

Although thyroid deficiencies (hypothyroidism) were recognized centuries ago and have long been treated by the consumption of animal thyroid glands, there is still much we do not know about how the thyroid works. Its relationship to brain sensitivities, for example, is just now becoming apparent.

Classical hypothyroid symptoms include a tendency toward obesity; dry, rough skin; brittle, dry hair that falls out easily and can become prematurely gray; a loss of the outer third of the eyebrows; increased sensitivity to cold; increased susceptibility to bruising; and a slowing of mental and physical activities. We believe that a tendency to develop multiple brain sensitivities can be added to this list. Of course, not everyone who has hypothyroidism suffers all these symptoms. And it is also possible for someone who exhibits none of the classical symptoms to have brain sensitivities due to a lack of thyroid hormone. Mr. G, one of our early cases in this use of thyroid, is a good example.

THE THIN MAN

When Mr. G initially came to us, he suffered from depression and anxiety and could barely function. After six years of psychotherapy, he had improved to the point where he was no longer neurotically dependent on his family; he was working on his own and had developed a number of creative talents that had been lying dormant. However, he also had multiple brain sensitivities to food which were complicating his life. Although he no longer lacked drive, he did lack energy and had to drag himself around most of the time. He had trouble waking up in the morning no matter how long he slept, and he was constantly catching colds and flu.

We traced many of his symptoms to the fact that Mr. G was sensitive to almost everything he ate. He improved markedly on a fast, but he was so thin and had so much trouble gaining weight that continuing a fast was out of the question. We put him on a strict rotation diet, but he was unable to eliminate the sensitizing foods for the initial period of abstinence because doing so would have meant going on a prolonged fast.

We had heard of the use of thyroid in the treatment of brain sensitivities, and we had our own clinical evidence to prove that it worked. In Mr. G's case, however, we were reluctant to use it. He certainly didn't have a classical medical history suggestive of hypothyroidism; his laboratory tests indicated normal thyroid blood levels, and he was so thin that we were almost certain he could not be a victim of hypothyroidism. When all else had failed, we discussed the situation with Mr. G. He was eager to try the treatment. We started him on a low dose of thyroid, and within a week he was able to eat with impunity most of the foods he had not been able to eat before. By the end of three more weeks on thyroid he was able to eat everything without any signs of sensitivity, and he gave up his rotation diet altogether.

It has been over three years now since Mr. G started taking thyroid. He has had no ill effects from it; he has had no further sensitivity reactions; he is living an active, normal life. And he has even gained some weight.

Blood tests that accurately measure the level of thyroid hormone in the blood do exist. Since the range of a normal concentration of thyroid is known, you might assume—as many physicians do—that determining whether or not a patient has hypothyroidism would be a simple matter of drawing a blood sample and comparing it to the normal range. If the results fall below the normal range, the patient has hypothyroidism; if they fall within the normal range, he doesn't. Unfortunately, this type of reasoning contains a basic error; as a result, many patients who actually have hypothyroidism are being misdiagnosed as normal —and often, if their symptoms persist, as neurotic.

The error lies in comparing an individual to a statistical range, and it is made over and over again in the interpretation of many different laboratory tests. The normal range of a test is usually determined as follows: A group of apparently normal people are chosen and the test is performed. The normal range is defined as the values between which 95 percent of these test results fall. But even if your score falls within that range, it doesn't necessarily mean that you are normal. Only the score that is normal for you would indicate whether or not you are hypothyroid. For example, if the normal range for a thyroid test is 5 to 12 and your normal value is 10, a result of 6 would mean you are hypothyroid, even though 6 falls within the normal range.

This, unfortunately, is not the only reason the blood test can be misunderstood. The thyroid test measures the amount of thyroid in the blood, but thyroid actually works in the tissues—the blood is merely the highway on which the hormone travels from the thyroid gland to its target areas in the body. Knowing how much thyroid is in the blood doesn't necessarily tell you how much is reaching its goal. Thus, if the levels of thyroid in the tissues are not adequate, you may still have hypothyroidism despite normal levels of thyroid in the blood.

Another, often more reliable, test for determining your thyroid function exists, and it can be performed at home (see Appendix 3, p. 167).

Thyroid hormone tablets that can correct the symptoms of hypothyroidism are available by prescription. You will therefore need the cooperation of a physician, who will monitor possible side effects, adjust the thyroid dosage, and determine the best form of thyroid for you.

Thyroid hormone works in conjunction with vitamin B complex and vitamin C. We have found that if patients are deficient in thyroid, vitamin B complex, and vitamin C, giving them the vitamins without thyroid can result in a worsening of their hypothyroid condition. Similarly, giving them thyroid without vitamin B complex and vitamin C may result in symptoms of hyperthyroidism (overactive thyroid), such as tremulousness or palpitations. Under these circumstances physicians are apt to make the error of discontinuing the thyroid hormone (or, in the first instance, the vitamins), when in fact the patient needs all three. Giving them together could eliminate the hypo or hyperthyroid reactions.

The Thymus Gland The thymus is an endocrine gland located under the breastbone. Until recently the predominant medical view was that, in adults, the thymus becomes a vestigial organ—an organ with no function. Because the thymus gland is large in children and tends to shrink and shrivel up after puberty, it was assumed that the gland was tied to growth and maturation and that, after puberty, it no longer had a role to play.

However, recent scientific research has verified what some clinicians have been saying all along: that the adult thymus is far from a vestigial organ. It does shrink after puberty, but it continues to function throughout life.

The role of the thymus that has most recently been getting the most scientific attention is its stimulatory effect on key elements of the body's defense system. This immune mechanism, which plays a role in protecting the body from disease, is also involved in some sensitivity reactions. Our clinical experience over the past year or two has left little doubt that the thymus gland is a key factor in the development and severity of many brain sensitivities.

We have attempted to stimulate the thymus by using raw extracts of thymus tissue, a product that is available in tablet form at some health food stores and pharmacies. Frequently these tablets appear to be effective in overcoming or reducing brain sensitivities. The dosage of this extract does need to be carefully adjusted and readjusted for the best results; and because the extract can sometimes interfere with thyroid functioning, the relationship between the thymus and the thyroid glands needs to be carefully monitored. For these reasons treatment with thymus extract should be carried out under the supervision of a physician experienced in these areas.

Other Hormonal Glands   The endocrine glands are all integrally related and function best when they are in balance with one another; a malfunction in any one of them can lead directly or indirectly to brain sensitivities. Two of the other endocrine glands that are often directly involved in sensitivity reactions are the adrenal and the gonadal glands.

The adrenal glands, which sit atop the kidneys, are often called the stress glands. Poor functioning of the adrenal glands is often a major factor in lowering our threshold for a sensitivity reaction. The gonadal glands, or sex glands, can also malfunction and lower the sensitivity threshold. This is particularly obvious in women whose sensitivities are worse during certain phases of their menstrual cycle and better during other phases. (It is also not unusual for women to first develop sensitivities during or after a pregnancy or around menopause.)

Laboratory tests to evaluate the function of these glands have the same shortcomings as the tests for thyroid production. Problems of hormone-producing glands should be corrected under a doctor's care.

Often, mild endocrine problems of this nature can be corrected by extracts of raw animal glands. The use of these extracts is not yet widely accepted in traditional medical circles, where it is believed that digestion destroys the extracts' usefulness. There is some scientific evidence, however, that animal tissue extracts can affect specific organs of the human body. Experiments have shown that when radioactively labeled extracts from liver are fed to an animal, they concentrate in the animal's liver. Likewise, extracts of lung concentrate in the animal's lungs, and so on for each organ of the body. Clinical experience has also found these extracts to be effective when taken orally—especially if they are chewed or sucked.

Since these substances are food extracts, they can be obtained without a prescription. However, they should be used with care. The choice of a particular raw tissue extract, dosage, frequency of use, and interaction with other glands are all factors that have to be taken into account by a physician.

Hypoglycemia (Low Blood Sugar)   Although it is not specifically an endocrine disease, the condition of hypoglycemia may be caused by one or more hormonal disturbances. Hypoglycemia, which is itself a controversial subject, can be intimately related to brain sensitivities in two ways. First, many cases of hypoglycemia are actually examples of a sensitivity to sugar, to foods from which sugar is derived (corn, sugar cane or beets, for example), or to other foods that can lower blood sugar. Second, low blood sugar leads to a lower sensitivity threshold. Many symptoms connected with sensitivities clear up completely when hypoglycemia is controlled or corrected.

Blood sugar drops as a result of the action of insulin: an overproduction of insulin can lead to an excessive blood sugar drop. Although insulin-secreting tumors do account for a small percentage of cases of hypoglycemia, most cases are of the reactive variety. In one form of reactive hypoglycemia the blood sugar remains normal until the individual does something to rapidly raise his blood sugar. In reaction to this sudden rise, the pancreas oversecretes insulin, and this backlash results in a below-normal blood sugar level.

Because blood sugar or glucose is the body's primary source of energy, the level of sugar in the blood is of critical importance. Blood sugar is so necessary that when it drops below a certain level, we should expect a wide range of symptoms capable of affecting *any* part of the body—and particularly the central nervous system, which is most sensitive to drops in glucose level. Ironically, it is this very range of symptoms that has been a major factor in the controversy surrounding hypoglycemia. Traditional medicine traces a physical problem to a specific symptom or set of symptoms. When we encounter a problem such as hypoglycemia that can cause almost any symptom, we tend to doubt the validity of the problem. (For a discussion on the determination of hypoglycemia, see Appendix 3, pp. 167–168.)

Hypoglycemia can be successfully treated by a nutritional approach. The key points in this type of treatment are avoidance of substances that cause blood sugar to rise rapidly, proper diet, and nutritional supplements.

The most commonly used substances capable of shooting your blood sugar level up are sugar itself, alcohol, caffeine (found in coffee, tea, cola and chocolate) and tobacco. People with hypoglycemia have a tendency to get hooked on one or more of these substances, which they use to bolster their falling blood sugar. Although such remedies can yield temporary relief, they set up a vicious cycle that perpetuates and in the long run worsens the condition. A key step in the treatment of hypoglycemia is, therefore, the elimination of sugar, alcohol, caffeine and nicotine. Elimination of these substances is also called for in cases where the drop in blood sugar is due to malfunctioning of the glands (adrenal, pancreas, pituitary) that produce hormones that raise blood sugar.

A second key factor in the treatment of hypoglycemia is regulating the types of foods you do eat. The diet most widely used for this purpose is the high-protein, low-carbohydrate diet originally prescribed for hypoglycemia by Dr. Seale Harris in 1924 and advocated by Dr. Carlton Fredericks. Another dietary approach more popular in Europe and advocated in this country by Dr. Paavo Airola is the low-protein, high-complex carbohydrate (such as grains, fruits and vegetables) diet. Both diets eliminate refined carbohydrates; in our experience they are both effective. However, there are individuals who do better with one than with the other. It is best to determine the type of diet, amount of food intake, and frequency of meals in consultation with a nutritionally oriented physician. This is also true when it comes to the third aspect in the treatment program—nutritional supplements.

The use of nutritional supplements—as well as injectable adrenal cortical extract (ACE) in selected cases—to correct hypoglycemia has much clinical evidence to support it. The specific supplements and their dosages need to be geared to the individual. To this treatment program we usually add exercise and stress reduction.

NUTRITION, EXERCISE AND STRESS

Whether or not you have hypoglycemia, the overall state of your health—and with it your ability to resist and overcome brain sensitivities—will greatly depend on the general level of your nutrition, your pattern of exercise, and your ability to cope with stress. Inadequate nutrition and poor physical conditioning give sensitivities a chance to flourish, while excessive stress allows them to practically walk into your life. The simple use of sound principles of nutrition, exercise and stress reduction in your daily life is often enough to relieve the symptoms your sensitivities cause.

There are scores of self-help books on the market that deal with multiple aspects of stress, exercise and nutrition (see Bibliography), and it is not our purpose to recapitulate them. But certain facets apply directly to sensitivities. Let's examine some general principles for treating and perhaps curing brain sensitivities.

Nutrition Staying well-nourished means supplying the

body with the proper amounts of all the ingredients it needs. These requirements vary greatly from individual to individual. Unfortunately, many of us are undernourished without realizing it, even though we have plenty to eat and carry around a lot of weight to prove it. Undernourishment doesn't mean that we don't eat enough food, but that we don't eat enough of the right foods.

The responsibility lies partly with our society and culture, partly with us. Our society has slowly changed the nature of food itself —by growing it with chemical fertilizers, freezing it, canning it, drying it, pickling it, preserving it with chemicals, and spraying it with insecticides. Through methods such as these we have managed to produce enough food for all of us to eat, but we have sacrificed quality for quantity.

We cannot turn back the hands of the clock and return all farmlands to a process of natural growth and harvest without making radical changes in our cultural pattern. But what we as individuals can do is to ensure that the foods we eat and the nutritional supplements we take are as free of toxic substances as possible and that they provide us with a full and complete assortment of the things we need to stay healthy. And that is something very few people do.

What are some of the problems we have to contend with in our search for health and nutrition?

About 70 percent of all our food is now processed or treated with chemicals to, among other things, reduce spoilage or to improve its physical appearance. Processing brings about a loss of nutrients—crucial vitamins, minerals, enzymes, and other elements. It can also damage the food's protein content. Researchers have found that the act of canning or freezing foods destroys as much as 90 percent of vitamin B-6, as well as large amounts of other vitamins.

The milling of wheat to produce white flour robs the grain of most of its vitamin E, as well as large amounts of its magnesium, calcium and protein. What milling leaves behind is mainly starch. The "highly nutritious" commercial bread that is found in supermarkets has had some vitamins and iron artificially added to it;

unfortunately, the additions do not make up for the elements lost during milling.

Not only are the foods we eat often deficient in the nutrients we need, but they have also been contaminated with toxic heavy minerals, such as lead (via automobile exhaust and industrial pollution) and mercury (found in fish as a result of water pollution from industrial plants). These toxic minerals can actually interfere with the normal functioning of our bodies and predispose us to brain sensitivities. A recent scientific article indicated that, as a group, children with learning disabilities had more of the toxic minerals lead and cadmium in their hair than did a group of normal children.

Tests involving hair, urine and blood can detect toxic amounts of these heavy metals, as well as deficiencies of essential minerals (see Appendix 3, pp. 166–168). Where minerals are deficient, they can be replaced by oral supplements. Toxic levels of heavy metals can be removed from the body by a treatment process known as chelation therapy, in which certain substances bind the metals and eliminate them from the body. In milder cases, oral supplements of certain nutrients such as vitamin C or sodium alginate can function as chelating agents. For more severe cases, chelating drugs like BAL or EDTA may need to be injected.

Nutrients do not work alone but, rather, function together as a team. When they are all present, they help us stay at our best. But when one is missing, the entire organism can suffer. It is well known that the lack of even a single major nutrient can cause a severely disabling disease or even death. (For example, scurvy, that dread of ancient sailors, was caused by a dearth of vitamin C in their diets.) But what most people don't realize is that a small but chronic shortage of one or more nutrients, which may not actually be enough to create a classically recognized deficiency syndrome, may lead to many health problems, including the development of brain sensitivities.

Those people who have a *vitamin dependency* condition have an additional reason to take supplementary vitamins. Unlike a vitamin deficiency, which you can correct by taking relatively small amounts of the deficient vitamin, a vitamin dependency indicates an ongoing dependency on relatively large doses of a particular vitamin in order to function normally. Two of the more common vitamin dependencies are those of niacin (vitamin B-3) and pyridoxine (vitamin B-6). A vitamin dependency condition can lead to brain sensitivities. Large doses of the appropriate vitamins can be used to treat the dependency and reduce the brain sensitivities.

Fortunately, there are ways we can correct deficiencies, prevent sensitivities, and pave the way to better health. Although it is impossible to describe the ideal diet for everyone, individual differences among people being too great, we can offer a set of generalizations.

1. Eat whole foods rather than foods that have been fragmented or processed. Whole-grain breads are healthier than white bread; brown rice is preferable to processed white rice. (A study by Weston Price in the 1930s demonstrated this dramatically. Price did a survey of several relatively primitive cultures. He found that when the people exchanged their native food for the processed food of the "civilized" world, both their dental and their general health deteriorated drastically.)

2. Food grown in soil fertilized biologically and naturally is superior to food grown in depleted soil that has been replenished by chemical fertilizers.

3. Foods containing artificial and chemical preservatives or additives should be avoided whenever possible. Read labels carefully. (Bear in mind, however, that although labeling laws are improving, in some circumstances the labeling laws are inadequate, and certain substances may be added to the product without being declared on the label.)

4. Fresh food is generally better than frozen food, which is better than canned food. In a 1946 study that compared the effects on cats of raw milk and raw meat with those of pasteurized milk and cooked meat, Francis Pottinger found that the cats raised only on the processed, cooked food developed degenerative diseases such as arthritis, allergies and pneumonia. These conditions became worse with each succeeding generation until, after four generations, the cats could no longer reproduce. In contrast,

the animals on the raw diet remained healthy and continued to reproduce.

Cooking can deplete food of some of its vital elements, such as vitamins, minerals and enzymes. Many foods (particularly fruits and the majority of vegetables) are also easier to digest in their raw states. As great a percentage as possible of the food you eat (vegetables, fruits, nuts, seeds and carefully inspected dairy products) should be in raw natural form.

5. Hydrogenated fats are vegetable oils to which hydrogen atoms have been added in the laboratory to make them solid. These fats (such as margarine) are not biological and, in our opinion, can be harmful to the body. Although animal fats (such as butter) should not be eaten excessively, we favor them over hydrogenated fats.

6. Try to include nuts and seeds in your diet. Sunflower seeds, pumpkin seeds, almonds and sesame seeds all contain complete protein. In addition, sprouting seeds are an economical and efficient source of nutrition (see Appendix 4).

7. Animal-protein meats, fish and poultry should be eaten in moderation. If you can, obtain meats that are relatively free from additives and pesticides.

8. Remember that you may be sensitive to your drinking water or to the concentrations of additives such as fluoride and chlorine contained in most communities' water. If you drink bottled spring water, try to get it in glass, not plastic, jugs. As a rule, it is a good idea to drink six to eight glasses of water every day.

9. Eat slowly, in an unhurried atmosphere, and chew the food well.

10. Eat only when you are hungry.

11. Diets that are high in fat (fats accounting for more than 35 percent of the calories consumed) tend to irritate blood vessels and increase sensitivity to foods. Consequently, we recommend that dietary fat content be kept at low levels (somewhere between 10 percent and 25 percent of the total number of calories).

12. Supplement your diet with vitamins, minerals and other nutrients. Check with a specialist—physician or nutritionist—who can help you arrange a supplement program geared to your

individual needs. In our experience, "natural" vitamins extracted from foods with minimal processing are usually more effective than synthetic ones. This may be because they retain elements of the food from which they are derived, which may catalyze or augment their effect.

Some people can, however, develop sensitivities to vitamins. Certain preparations of synthetic vitamin C, for example, are made through an enzymatic process from corn glucose, and people who are sensitive to corn can develop symptoms when they take that form of vitamin C. Similarly, some brands of natural vitamin E are extracted from cereal grains, and individuals sensitive to these grains can react to that vitamin E. These individuals may be able to safely tolerate synthetic vitamin E or natural vitamin E from another source.

13. Do not overeat. Excesses of any food, no matter how wholesome, will add toxicity to your body.

14. Whenever possible, infants should be breast fed. Unquestionably, one of the major reasons for the widespread occurrence of allergies (especially to milk) in children and later in adults is the feeding of cow's milk or other formulas to infants before their digestive systems can handle this type of food. Breast milk is the perfect food for infants and is strongly recommended for the benefit of both child and mother.

Exercise   As important as good nutrition is, appropriate exercise is, in our opinion, even more important. In fact, if you have to choose between eating well without exercise and eating "junk" food with a good exercise program, you will in all likelihood be healthier with the latter choice. Fortunately, one is rarely forced to make such a choice and so can take advantage of the fact that a balanced combination of nutrition and exercise is one of the best hedges against symptoms of brain sensitivity.

There are three major types of exercises:

1. Exercises that stimulate the cardiovascular system, such as jogging, biking and swimming.

2. Stretching and loosening exercises, such as yoga.

3. Exercises that stimulate the "Chi" or life energy system (described in Chapter Five), such as Tai-Chi. Tai-Chi is an an-

cient Chinese dancelike exercise done in slow motion, which has beneficial effects on the body and mind as well as a stimulating effect on the life energy system (comparable to the effect of jogging on the cardiovascular system).

Ideally, one should take advantage of all three of these approaches. It is, of course, a good idea to check with a physician before undertaking an exercise program, particularly if it is strenuous.

Stress   In Chapter Seven we discussed the role of negative stress in producing and aggravating brain sensitivities. Although stress is an inevitable part of most of our lives, there is much we can do to change our response to that stress so as to minimize its impact.

Any of the pertinent treatments we have discussed will strengthen your resistance to stress. In addition, specific techniques are available—some centuries old, some relatively new— to help you relax and remain calm even in the face of considerable stress.

Following are some of these approaches:

1. *Meditation.* There are many forms of meditation available today, no one of which is inherently better than the others. If there is a particular form of meditation that feels right for you, you will probably get more from it than from another. All of them help you to relax.

2. *Progressive relaxation exercises.* These are exercises that progressively relax the voluntary muscles of the body in order to achieve a state of deep relaxation.

3. *Breathing techniques.* The quality of our breathing determines in large part how tense or how relaxed we feel. Most people do not breathe properly. You can learn breathing techniques in most yoga classes; also see the Bibliography for books specifically on breathing.

4. *Hypnotic techniques.* Under the guidance of an experienced and reputable practitioner, you can learn how to use self-hypnosis to minimize the harmful effects of stress.

5. *Biofeedback training.* This method makes use of biofeedback machines that can help you learn how to control functions of your body that are ordinarily not under voluntary control (such as

blood pressure and pulse rate). You can learn to relax your muscles, increase skin temperature, or produce an alpha brain wave rhythm, all of which promote a state of relaxation.

6. *Autogenic training.* This approach is also concerned with helping you gain control over functions of the body not usually under voluntary control—particularly those that relate to the homeostatic mechanisms of the body (those mechanisms that keep the body in balance and maintain its stability). Unlike biofeedback training, autogenic training utilizes no machines. Control is achieved completely through mind training, using a specific series of structured mental exercises that, among other benefits, can lead to deep states of relaxation.

7. *Martial art forms.* Martial art training can be external, internal, or a combination of both. The external system primarily teaches the art of fighting. The internal system de-emphasizes fighting and, instead, promotes internal strength, health and relaxation through exercise.

8. *Special forms of physical exercise.* Psychocalisthenic programs and bioenergetic exercises involve both the mind and the body. Books describing specific physical exercises drawn from these systems are listed in the Bibliography.

These techniques can also alleviate many psychological stresses, but forms of emotional illness do exist that require some form of psychological or psychiatric intervention.

OTHER ECOLOGICAL FACTORS

A number of other physical factors in our environment appear to affect our feelings of well-being and may contribute to the development of brain sensitivities. Three of the most promising areas for research and clinical application concern light, electrical charges in the atmosphere, and temperature.

Light In his book *Health and Light,* John Ott tells us that indirect light from the sun's rays is necessary for optimal health. Artificial lighting and wearing glass lenses may contribute to a wide variety of conditions such as fatigue, headaches and hyperactivity in children.

Consequently, we recommend that people expose themselves to *indirect* outdoor sunlight as often as possible. *(Warning: looking at the sun directly can be extremely harmful and can lead to blindness!)* If you need to wear lenses, full spectrum CR 39 plastic lenses should be used, as these do not cut off the beneficial ultraviolet rays of the sun. Certain indoor lights that more closely approximate the sun's rays than do ordinary fluorescent or incandescent bulbs are now also available.

Electricity in the Air Research indicates that the air we breathe is permeated with extremely small amounts of electrically charged particles called ions. These ions may be either positively or negatively charged. The negative ions that predominate after a rainstorm contribute to one's sense of well-being. On the other hand, the positive ions that are present in higher amounts on hot, heavy, humid days contribute to one's sense of discomfort.

Electrically produced negative ions have been successfully used in the treatment of burns and respiratory conditions. People appear to function well when the ionic concentration of the air we breathe is 1,000 to 2,000 ions per cubic centimeter of air, with negative ions predominating slightly. A variety of man-made factors, including pollution, central air conditioning, forced-air heating systems, and automobiles, tend to be harmful in two ways. They significantly reduce the total ionic concentration in the air, and they increase the proportion of positive ions to negative ions. Both of these effects are detrimental to at least a certain percentage of the population.

Clinical experiences in Israel, Germany, and Russia indicate that these deleterious effects may be counteracted by negative-ion generator machines. Although such devices have not yet been approved for any therapeutic purpose by the Federal Food and Drug Administration in the United States, they can be sold as long as no therapeutic claims are made for them. As of this writing, desk models about the size of a lamp are available in the United States for about seventy-five dollars from a variety of distributors.

Temperature Allergists have known for many years that allergic reactions may be affected or caused by extreme temperatures.

Reactions may occur in response to weather changes or to hot or cold foods. One way of building resistance to temperature changes is to alternate warm and cold showers back and forth a few times, allowing thirty seconds for each change in temperature. Gradually increase the extremes of temperature.

BEYOND BODY AND MIND

We believe that there is a spiritual essence to each of us. Unfortunately, this aspect of our being, which is so vitally involved in our states of illness and health, is the one least often addressed by the medical profession today. It is, in our opinion, a grievous and unnecessary lack. Our cultural emphasis on goal-oriented and materialistic values does much to numb our awareness of our own spirituality. Many of us give it lip service, but few of us feel it as a living, warm, vital part of ourselves. Practical techniques such as specialized forms of breathing, movement and meditation can help us to reconnect in a meaningful way with the spiritual part of our being. We have seen brain sensitivities and other physical problems disappear when people make this kind of reconnection. Not only can self-healing occur (who has not heard of spontaneous remissions or miraculous recoveries even in the face of death?), but one's entire life can be enriched.

We have presented both specific and general therapeutic measures for the treatment of brain sensitivities. In so doing, we have had to discuss them separately. In actual practice, however, we generally draw freely from them and combine them, when appropriate, to meet the needs of the person with whom we are working.

It is our belief that when someone becomes ill, the illness manifests itself on every level of that person's being. If we choose to look at that individual from a psychological point of view, we will see the manifestation of the illness on a mental level. If we choose to look at that same individual from a biochemical point of view, we will see the manifestation of that illness on a metabolic level. These, as well as other levels, such as physical, energetic (Chi) and spiritual, all coexist. Rather than representing opposing views of what the illness is, they complement one another, enabling us to see and deal with the illness from a number of different perspectives. Each of these perspectives offers the potential of another clinical tool with which to combat the illness.

If we confine ourselves to only one level of treatment, some people will undoubtedly respond better to a biochemical approach, some to a psychological approach, and so forth. However, if we take a holistic view and are prepared to give and receive help on more than one level, we can generally move more effectively toward the goal of optimum health. This is as true of treating a brain sensitivity as it is of treating any other malfunction of the body.

In advocating that brain sensitivity be seriously considered in the evaluation and treatment of a wide range of emotional problems, we are not attempting to discredit or to replace other valid therapeutic forms; rather, we are adding to them. It is in this spirit that we have incorporated the principles of brain sensitivity into our work, and it is in this spirit that we have offered to share what we have learned about brain sensitivities.

APPENDICES

APPENDIX 1:
Signs and Symptoms That May Indicate Sensitivity Reactions

The following list indicates the possible scope of the food-chemical sensitivity problem.

1. *Central Nervous System*
   Depression
   Drowsiness
   Fatigue
   Learning disorders
   Minimal brain dysfunction
   Anxiety
   Insomnia
   Hyperactivity
   Poor memory
   Poor concentration
   Feelings of unreality
   Personality changes
   Withdrawal
   Angry outbursts
   Hallucinations
   Delusions
   Dizziness
   Vertigo
   Hot flashes
   Confusion
   Headaches of all kinds (tension, vascular, migraines)
   Seizure disorders

2. *Eyes and Vision*
    Sensitivity to light
    Blurred vision
    Double vision
    Dyslexia (difficulty in reading)
    Itching
    Burning
    Pain
    Heavy feeling

3. *Ears and Hearing*
    Itching
    Full (blocked feeling)
    Earache
    Hearing loss
    Ringing
    Increased sensitivity to sound

4. *Sinuses, Nose and Sense of Smell*
    Stuffy
    Itching
    Sneezing
    Reduced sense of smell
    Increased sense of smell
    Obstruction
    Sinus pain and tenderness

5. *Mouth and Throat*
    Sores in mouth
    Swollen gums
    Difficulty in swallowing
    Increased or decreased salivation
    Bad taste in mouth
    Sore throat
    Hoarseness
    Swelling in throat

6. *Lungs*
    Difficulty in breathing
    Asthma (wheezing)
    Coughing
    Hyperventilation (rapid overbreathing)

7. *Gastro-Intestinal and Abdomen*
   Bloating
   Nausea
   Reduced appetite
   Increased appetite
   Abdominal pain
   Cramps
   Diarrhea
   Spastic colon
   Mucous colitis
   Increased belching
   Increased flatus
   Hyperacidity
   Itchy anus

8. *Heart and Blood Vessels*
   Chest pain
   Angina
   Palpitations
   Rapid heartbeat (pulse)
   Extra beats (premature atrial contractions [PACs] or premature
      ventricular contractions [PVCs])
   Generalized swelling
   Inflammation of veins
   Inflammation of arteries

9. *Muscles and Joints*
   Muscle cramps
   Muscle spasms
   Muscle tremors or jerks
   Muscle weakness
   Muscle stiffness
   Achy joints
   Stiff joints
   Swollen joints
   Myositis (inflammation of muscles)
   Arthritis (inflammation of joints)

10. *Urinary—Genital*
    Frequency of urination
    Bedwetting

Urgent need to urinate (pressure)
Painful urination
Need to urinate during the night
Painful periods (menses)
Heavy periods (menses)
Irregular periods (menses)
Increase or decrease in sexual drive

11. *Skin*
Local itching
Generalized itching
Hives
Pallor (white color)
Increase or decrease in perspiring
Acne
Eczema
Many skin lesions

12. *Blood*
Anemia (reduced red blood cells)
Leukopenia (reduced white blood cells)
Thrombocytopenia (reduced platelets)
Increase or decrease in clotting
Decreased immunity

APPENDIX 2:
Food Families
and the Rotation Diet

Prepared by Susan Shaw

First eliminate all foods that cause allergic reactions; then rotate the remaining foods on a four-day or a seven-day basis to ensure diversity in the diet. The following diets are based on a four-day and seven-day rotation cycle, respectively.

Ideally a food should be eaten only once a day. However, this is not always possible on a seven-day rotation plan, and occasionally it becomes difficult on a four-day schedule. Be aware that repeating foods vertically (within the same day) may or may not produce an allergic reaction. If a sensitivity does develop as a result of repeating a food within the same day, note this reaction and avoid eating that food more than once daily in the future.

Menus are flexible, provided that meals are made from the families listed for that day. Also, lunch entrees and side dishes may be eaten at the evening meal, and vice versa.

FAMILIES

In order to prevent cross-sensitization, all foods are rotated according to family groupings. For example, members of the large mustard family, which appear on Day I of the four-day rotation diet (mustard, greens, turnip, broccoli, radish, cauliflower, etc.), do not reappear until Day I of the second cycle, or four days later. In the seven-day rotation diet, these families are spaced at seven-day intervals.

RECIPES

Any recipes you may wish to use should conform to the rotation plan. The lists of food families for each day may be used to provide alternative menus. Recipe ingredients that do not conform to the food families listed for a given day should be omitted, and other ingredients should be substituted.

CALORIES

The caloric content of each of the sample menus listed subsequently (for both the four- and the seven-day rotation diets) is approximately 2,500 calories. If fewer or more calories are desired, appropriate adjustments should be made.

HERBS

In the rotation diets, herbs are grouped according to families. They may be used for seasonings, sauces or salad dressings. Herbs should be strictly rotated, just as the other plant families are rotated. In many instances, herbs belong to larger plant families, such as the parsley family on Day II of the four-day rotation diet, which includes dill, cumin, coriander, caraway and anise. A great variety of fresh and dried herbs can be found in health food stores and specialty herb shops.

FRUITS AND VEGETABLES

Some people develop excessive gas when they eat certain foods such as fruits and vegetables at the same meal. The sample diets that follow do not take this into account and when necessary will have to be changed accordingly.

FISH, MOLLUSKS, CRUSTACEANS

Most fish, mollusks and crustaceans are classified as separate, individual food families. For example, oysters are considered a family, clams another family, lobster another family, and so on.

The fish families that include more than one type of fish are: salmon, herring, cod, mackerel, flounder, whiting, pompano, pike, buffalo, bass, black bass and yellow perch. All other fish (whitefish, carp, red snapper, etc.) are considered families in themselves. You may refer to the listings of fish, mollusks and crustaceans as they appear in their taxonomical groupings:

MOLLUSKS   *Scallops*
            Oysters
            Cockles
            Clams
            Abalone
            Snails
            Squid

CRUSTACEANS *Shrimp*
            Lobster
            Crab

FISH   *Sturgeon*
            Paddlefish
            Tarpon
            Herring   Herring, shad
            Anchovy
            Salmon   Salmon, trout
            Whitefish
            Smelt
            Pike (Northern)   Northern pike, muskellunge
            Buffalo   Buffalo, sucker
            Carp
            Catfish
            Common Eel
            Conger Eel
            Cod   Cod, haddock, pollack, tomcod, silver hake
            Mullet
            Bass   Striped bass, rockfish, spotted bass, black sea bass, grouper, hind, white perch
            Black Bass   Largemouth black bass, smallmouth black bass, spotted black bass, sunfish, pumpkinseed, bluegill
            Red Snapper
            Grunt
            Yellow Perch   Yellow perch, walleye, pike
            Bluefish
            Pompano   Pompano, amberjack, jack mackerel
            Dolphin Fish
            Whiting   Whiting, weakfish, croaker, freshwater drumfish
            Porgy
            Mackerel   Atlantic mackerel, Spanish mackerel, king mackerel, bluefish tuna, bonito, frigate mackerel, skipjack tuna
            Butterfish
            Flounder   Flounder, halibut
            Sole

Ocean Perch, Rosefish
Sea Robins, Sea Tags
Puffer

BIRDS (AVES)

Birds are also classified as separate, individual food families, with the exceptions of the duck and quail families, which include more than one member.

The taxonomical classification of birds includes the following families:

Duck   Mallard duck, greylag goose
Grouse
Quail   Quail, peafowl, pheasant, chicken, chicken eggs
Guinea Fowl
Turkey
Pigeon

SHOPPING GUIDELINES

The following foods may be purchased at a health food store or the health food section of a supermarket:

Honey Honey should be raw, unfiltered and unheated; in this state it provides enzymes, minerals and amino acids

Oils Oils such as sesame and olive should be cold-pressed, unrefined, and free of bleaching agents or preservatives

Dairy Products Dairy products such as cheese and butter should be obtained from raw milk (cow's or goat's milk) when available. (Processed cheese should be avoided.)

Sprouts Alfalfa and mung sprouts are generally available; some stores stock unusual sprouts such as lentils, chick-peas, wheat, and adzuki bean sprouts, which make a delicious addition to salads (see Appendix 4 for instructions on home sprouting)

Dried Fruits Dried fruits such as apricots, currants, apples, raisins, prunes, dates and figs should always be unsulphured

Nuts A variety of nuts, preferably raw, can be purchased in most stores: almonds, filberts, hazelnuts, cashews, pistachios, walnuts, beechnuts, pine nuts, macadamia nuts, hickory nuts

Nut Butters Delicious nut butters include almond butter, fresh peanut butter and cashew butter

Seeds Sesame seeds, sunflower seeds, squash and pumpkin seeds, psyllium, flaxseeds, chia

Seed Butters Sesame butter, sesame paste (tahini), sunflower butter

Fresh Juices Fresh juices such as carrot, carrot-celery, tomato, tomato-cucumber, green juices,* and fresh-squeezed citrus juices may be purchased or prepared at home. These juices are highly perishable, and it is best to drink them as soon as possible after they are squeezed

Nectars and Unsweetened Bottled Juices

Grains Wheat berries, brown rice, barley, rye and millet, buckwheat (kasha), bulgur, oats

Legumes Peas, lentils, mung beans, garbanzos (chick-peas), kidney and other dry beans, carob, alfalfa, licorice and soybeans

Soy Products Soy flour, soy sprouts, lecithin, soybean oil and tofu (bean curd)

---

*Juices made from green vegetables such as spinach, escarole, or green peppers. They may be mixed with other juices such as carrot juice for sweetening.

Four-Day Rotation Diet

FOOD FAMILIES: DAY 1

Pineapple   Pineapple
Palm   Coconut, date, date sugar
Citrus   Lemon, orange, grapefruit, lime, tangerine, kumquat, citron, tangelo, mandarin orange, mandarin tangerine
Buckwheat   Buckwheat, rhubarb
Mustard   Mustard, mustard greens, turnip, radish, horseradish, watercress, cabbage (red or white), kraut, Chinese (celery) cabbage, broccoli, cauliflower, Brussels sprouts, kale, collards, kohlrabi, rutabaga, Savoy cabbage
Beech   Filbert, hazelnut
Sweet Potato (Morning Glory) or Yam
Olive   Black or green olives
Myrtle   Allspice, cloves, guava, pimento
Ginseng   Ginseng root
Comfrey   Comfrey root, leaves
Bovid   Beef, veal, lamb, goat; dairy products (butter, cheese, cottage cheese, yogurt, kefir, buttermilk)
Salmon   Salmon, trout
Turkey

Tea   Comfrey, ginseng
Oil   Butter, coconut oil, olive oil
Sweetener   Date sugar, orange blossom honey*
Juice   Juices (unsweetened) may be made from any of the fruits or vegetables listed above, including fresh comfrey

*Honey should be raw, unheated and unfiltered. If used today, honey should not be repeated on another day of the four-day rotation.

SAMPLE DIET: DAY 1

Breakfast   Orange juice (4 ounces)*
Fresh pineapple slices, orange slices (1 cup)
Bowl of buckwheat (kasha) cereal (⅓ cup dry) with 1 pat of but-
ter** and 1 teaspoon date sugar
Ginseng or comfrey tea

Snack   2 ounces filberts
4 or 5 dates

Lunch   1 glass (6 ounces) grapefruit juice*
3 ounces lean veal*** or fowl (turkey without skin)
½ cup steamed cauliflower with 1 ounce melted cheddar
½ cup baked sweet potato or yam with 1 pat of butter**
1 cup steamed greens (mustard, turnip, kale or collards)
6 to 8 green olives stuffed with pimentos
6 raw radishes
1 cup yogurt with 2 ounces shredded coconut

Snack   Tangerine or tangelo

Dinner   4 ounces broiled salmon or trout
or
4 ounces lean beef or lamb***
1 cup steamed Brussels sprouts or broccoli with 1 pat of butter**
1 cup steamed cabbage or kohlrabi
Salad:
½ cup shredded red cabbage
½ cup watercress
6 black olives
2 ounces cottage cheese**
Dressing:
1 tablespoon olive oil and ¼ lemon (juice)
½ cup mandarin oranges or guavas
1 glass (6 ounces) milk or buttermilk**

Bedtime   Comfrey tea

*Juice should be unsweetened (preferably fresh-squeezed).
**If possible, dairy products should be made from raw milk (available at health food
stores).
***Horseradish or mustard may be used as a sauce for meat.

FOOD FAMILIES: DAY 2

Banana   Banana, plantain, psyllium seed
Honeysuckle   Elderberry
Gooseberry   Currants, gooseberry
Heath (Blueberry)   Blueberry, huckleberry, cranberry, wintergreen
Grape   Grapes (all varieties), raisins
Holly   Pokeberry, bearberry, maté
Walnut   English walnut, black walnut, pecan, hickory nut, butternut
Goosefoot (Beet)   Beet, spinach, chard, lamb's-quarters (greens), sugar beet
Pedalium   Sesame seed, sesame paste (tahini), oil, sesame butter
Parsley   Carrot, parsnip, parsley, celery, celery seed, celeriac, anise, dill, fennel,
    cumin, coriander, caraway, chervil
Fungus   Mushroom, yeast
Beech   Beechnut, chestnut
Quail   Chicken, quail, peafowl, pheasant, chicken eggs
Flounder   Flounder, halibut
Cod   Cod, haddock, pollack, tomcod, silver hake
Prawn
Crayfish
Cockles
Clams
Mussels
Oysters
Scallops

Tea   Elderberry, blueberry, pokeberry, bearberry, fennel
Oil   Sesame seed oil
Sweetener   Beet sugar, clover honey (if honey was not used on another day of
    rotation)
Juice   Juices (unsweetened) can be made from any of the fruits or vegetables
    listed above

SAMPLE DIET: DAY 2

Breakfast   Grape juice (4 ounces, unsweetened)
Raisin and nut cereal*
1 sliced banana
Blueberry tea

Snack   Handful (1 ounce) of hickory nuts
1 cup of fresh blueberries

Lunch   4 ounces broiled fish (cod family), shellfish** or mushroom omelette
(2 eggs, without milk)
1 cup baked parsnips or plantains
1 cup steamed beets
Salad:
    1 cup raw spinach
    ½ cup raw chervil
    ½ cup mushrooms (sliced)
Dressing:
    1 tablespoon sesame oil and fresh dill
    ½ cup chestnut purée (sweetened with honey or 1 teaspoon beet
    sugar)
Fennel tea

Snack   Handful (1 ounce) of pecans
2 ounces currants***

Dinner   1 glass (8 ounces) fresh carrot juice with 1 to 2 ounces parsley or
spinach juice
4 ounces lean fowl† without skin, or fish (flounder, halibut), with
    ¼ cup cranberry sauce (sweetened with honey)
1 cup steamed Swiss chard or lamb's-quarters
1 cup steamed carrots with parsley
Salad:
    Celery and carrot sticks
    Raw fennel
    2 teaspoons tahini (sesame paste) or sesame butter and herbs
1 cup grapes

Bedtime   Elderberry tea

*Raisin and nut cereal: 2 ounces raisins and 3 ounces nuts (walnuts, pecans, hickory
nuts, butternuts, beechnuts; psyllium seeds), ground to make a fine cereal.
**Prawn, crayfish, clams, mussels, oysters, scallops, cockles.
***Dried fruits should be unsulphured (available at health food stores).
†Family: quail (chicken, quail, peafowl, pheasant, chicken eggs).

FOOD FAMILIES: DAY 3

Rose Strawberry, raspberry, blackberry, dewberry, loganberry, youngberry, boysenberry, rose hip

Apple Apple, pear, quince

Plum Plum, prune, cherry, peach, apricot, nectarine, almond, persimmon (ebony), wild cherry

Protea Macadamia nut

Conifer Pine nut

Flaxseed Flaxseed

Legume Black-eyed pea, carob (St.-John's-bread, locust bean), fava or broad bean (vetch), alfalfa, garbanzo (chick-pea), snap bean, goober, green pea, kidney bean (frijol), lentil, licorice, lima bean, mung bean, navy bean, peanut (and oil), pigeon pea, pinto bean, soybean, soy flour, lecithin, soybean oil, string bean, tamarind, wax bean, snowpea; sprouts (mung, soybean, chick-pea, lentil, alfalfa)

Grass (Cereal) Wheat, corn, rice, oats, barley, malt, rye, wild rice, millet, sorghum, molasses, bamboo shoots, cane; sprouts (wheat)

Lily Onion, garlic, asparagus, chive, leek, Bermuda onion, shallot, scallion, Spanish onion

Cypera Chinese water chestnut

Maranta Arrowroot

Ginger Ginger, turmeric

Iris Saffron (flower and seed)

Duck Mallard duck, greylag goose

Swine Pork, pork products

Crab

Lobster

Shrimp

Abalone

Snails

Squid

Sole Sole

Bass Striped bass, rockfish, spotted bass, black sea bass, grouper, hind, white perch

Black Bass Largemouth and smallmouth black bass, spotted black bass, sunfish, pumpkinseed, bluegill

---

Tea Rose hip, alfalfa, licorice root, berry

Oil Soybean, peanut, flaxseed

Sweetener Carob syrup, corn syrup, tupelo or wildflower honey (if honey was not used on another day of rotation), molasses, sorghum

Juice Juices (unsweetened) may be made from any of the fruits or vegetables listed above, including sprouts

SAMPLE DIET: DAY 3

Breakfast Apricot nectar (4 ounces)
Bowl of millet or oatmeal ($\frac{1}{3}$ cup dry) with 1 teaspoon molasses and 1 teaspoon ground flaxseed
$\frac{1}{3}$ cup prunes or dried apricots*
Rose hip or alfalfa tea

Snack 1 ounce macadamia nuts or pine nuts
1 apple

Lunch 4 ounces steamed shrimp, crabmeat or broiled fish**
2 cups Chinese vegetables sautéed with $\frac{1}{2}$ cup tofu (bamboo shoots, water chestnuts, scallions, onions, snowpeas, mung sprouts, soybean sprouts, fresh ginger, and with 1 tablespoon arrowroot starch for thickening
$\frac{1}{2}$ cup brown rice or wild rice
1 persimmon or pear
Rose hip tea

Snack 2 rice cakes with 2 teaspoons fresh peanut butter or handful (1 ounce) of raw almonds

Dinner 1 cup pea or lentil soup
4 ounces lean pork, broiled shellfish*** or broiled fish,** or 4 ounces broiled fowl† (without skin), or 6 ounces steamed squid, clams or mussels
Fresh corn on cob (1 ear) or $\frac{1}{2}$ cup pearl barley
1 cup steamed asparagus
Sprout salad:
   2 cups fresh sprouts (alfalfa, lentil, wheat, chick-pea or mung)
   $\frac{1}{4}$ cup chopped chives or shallots
Dressing:
   1 tablespoon soybean or peanut oil, fresh ginger, minced, and tamari (soy sauce)††
1 cup fresh strawberries

Bedtime Licorice tea

*Dried fruits should be unsulphured.
**Families: sole, bass or black bass.
***Families: lobster, abalone, squid, snail.
†Duck (mallard duck, greylag goose).
††Tamari (soy sauce) may be used for flavoring.

FOOD FAMILIES: DAY 4

Mulberry   Mulberry, fig, breadfruit
Pawpaw   Pawpaw, papaya, papain
Custard   Cherimoya
Gourd   Watermelon, cantaloupe, winter melon and other melons, pumpkin, cucumber, zucchini, squash; pumpkin and squash seeds
Cashew   Cashew, pistachio, mango
Sapucaia   Brazil nut
Mallow   Okra, cottonseed
Potato   Potato, tomato, eggplant, red and green pepper, chili pepper, paprika, cayenne
Pepper   Black and white pepper, peppercorns
Aster   Lettuce, chicory, endive, escarole, artichoke, Jerusalem artichoke, dandelion, sunflower seeds and oil, tarragon, safflower oil, chamomile, goldenrod
Laurel   Avocado, cinnamon, bay leaf, sassafras, cassia buds or cassia bark
Nutmeg   Nutmeg, mace
Spurge   Tapioca
Orchid   Vanilla
Maple   Maple sugar and syrup
Mint   Basil, savory, sage, oregano, horehound, catnip, spearmint, peppermint, thyme, marjoram, lemon balm
Grouse
Guinea Fowl
Pigeon
Herring   Herring, shad
Whitefish
Mackerel   Mackerel, tuna, bonito
Porgy
Bluefish
Pompano   Pompano, amberjack, jack mackerel
Red Snapper
Whiting   Whiting, weakfish, croaker, freshwater drumfish
Sturgeon
Anchovy
Butterfish
Sardine

Tea   Mint, sassafras, papaya, chamomile
Oil   Cottonseed, sunflower seed, safflower oil
Sweetener   Maple sugar and syrup, avocado honey, sage honey (if honey was not used on another day of rotation)
Juice   Juices (unsweetened) may be made from any of the fruits or vegetables listed above, including tea herbs and melons

SAMPLE DIET: DAY 4

Breakfast   Papaya juice (4 ounces, unsweetened)
  1 cup fresh mango and papaya slices
  Fig and nut cereal* with 1 teaspoon maple syrup
  Papaya or chamomile tea
Snack   2 ounces pistachio nuts or sunflower seeds
  1 cup cherimoyas or ½ fresh papaya
Lunch   Fresh tomato juice (8 ounces) or tomato-cucumber juice
  3 ounces tuna, herring or sardines
  ½ cup baked squash (butternut or acorn)
  Salad:
    1 cup romaine or Boston lettuce
    ½ cucumber, sliced
    ½ zucchini, sliced
    3 or 4 Jerusalem artichokes, sliced
    ½ ripe avocado
  Dressing:
    1 tablespoon safflower oil and herbs (basil, thyme, tarragon or
      marjoram)
  Sassafras tea
Snack   ½ cantaloupe, small honeydew, casaba or other melon; 4 inch ×
    4 inch wedge of watermelon
Dinner   6 ounces fresh tomato juice
  4 ounces broiled or baked fish** or 4 ounces broiled fowl*** (with-
    out skin)
  1 medium baked potato
  1 cup stewed okra and eggplant with tomatoes
  Salad:
    6 artichoke hearts
    1 cup escarole and endive
    ½ cup dandelion leaves
    Red and green pepper slices
  Dressing:
    1 tablespoon sunflower seed oil, ½ avocado (mashed), herbs
  ½ cup tapioca (vanilla, sweetened with maple sugar)
Bedtime   Fennel or peppermint tea

*Fig and nut cereal: 2 ounces chopped figs and 2 ounces nuts and seeds (cashews, Brazil
nuts; sunflower seeds, pumpkin and squash seeds), ground to a fine cereal.
**Families: whitefish, mackerel, porgy, bluefish, pompano, red snapper, whiting, stur-
geon, butterfish.
***Grouse, guinea fowl or pigeon.

Seven-Day Rotation Diet

FOOD FAMILIES: DAY 1

Pineapple   Pineapple
Palm   Coconut, date, date sugar
Buckwheat   Buckwheat, rhubarb
Mustard   Mustard, mustard greens, turnip, radish, horseradish, watercress, cabbage (red or white), kraut, Chinese (celery) cabbage, broccoli, cauliflower, Brussels sprouts, kale, collards, kohlrabi, rutabaga, Savoy cabbage
Beech   Filbert, hazelnut
Comfrey   Comfrey leaves, root
Bovid   Beef, veal, lamb, goat; dairy products (butter, cheese, cottage cheese, yogurt, kefir, buttermilk)*
Salmon   Salmon, trout

Tea   Comfrey tea
Oil   Butter, coconut oil
Sweetener   Date sugar, clover honey** (if honey was not used on another day of the rotation)
Juice   Juices (unsweetened) may be made from any of the fruits or vegetables listed above, including fresh comfrey

*If possible, dairy products should be obtained from raw milk.
**Honey should be raw, unheated and unfiltered.

SAMPLE DIET: DAY 1

Breakfast 1 glass (4 ounces) pineapple-coconut juice*
Fresh pineapple slices (1 cup)
Bowl of buckwheat (kasha) cereal ($\frac{1}{3}$ cup dry) with 1 pat of butter and 1 teaspoon date sugar
1 glass (6 ounces) buttermilk or kefir**
Comfrey tea

Snack Handful (1 ounce) filberts or hazelnuts

Lunch 1 glass (6 ounces) milk
3 ounces lean veal
1 cup baked turnips or rutabagas with 1 pat of butter, horseradish sauce
1 cup steamed collards or kale
$\frac{1}{2}$ cup steamed Brussels sprouts
6 to 8 raw radishes

Snack 1 cup yogurt with 1 tablespoon shredded coconut and 1 teaspoon date sugar

Dinner 4 ounces broiled salmon or trout or 4 ounces lean beef or lamb (mustard sauce)
1 cup broccoli or cauliflower (steamed) with 1 ounce melted cheddar
1 cup steamed mustard or turnip greens
Salad:
$\frac{1}{2}$ cup shredded red cabbage
$\frac{1}{2}$ cup chopped watercress
2 ounces cottage cheese
4 dates*** stuffed with coconut
Comfrey tea

Bedtime Comfrey tea

*Juice should be unsweetened.
**If possible, dairy products should be obtained from raw milk (available in health food stores).
***Dried fruit should be unsulphured.

FOOD FAMILIES: DAY 2

Citrus   Lemon, orange, grapefruit, lime, tangerine, kumquat, citron, tangelo, mandarin orange, mandarin tangerine

Rose   Strawberry, raspberry, blackberry, dewberry, loganberry, youngberry, boysenberry, rose hip

Grass (Cereal)   Wheat, corn, rice, wild rice, oats, barley, malt, rye, millet, sorghum, molasses, bamboo shoots, cane; wheat sprouts

Lily   Onion, garlic, asparagus, chive, leek, Bermuda onion, shallot, scallion, Spanish onion

Flaxseed   Flaxseed

Fungus   Mushroom, yeast

Iris   Saffron (flower and seed)

Orchid   Vanilla

Spurge   Tapioca

Ginger   Ginger, turmeric

Duck   Mallard duck, greylag goose

Sardine

Sturgeon

Paddlefish

Tarpon

Herring   Herring, shad

Anchovy

Whitefish

Smelt

———————————

Tea   Rose hip, saffron, blackberry

Oil   Corn, flaxseed

Sweetener   Orange blossom honey (if honey was not used on another day of the rotation), molasses, sorghum

Juice   Juices (unsweetened) may be made from any of the fruits or vegetables listed above

SAMPLE DIET: DAY 2

Breakfast 1 glass (6 ounces) fresh orange juice*
1 cup strawberries or blackberries
Bowl of millet or oatmeal cereal (⅓ cup dry)
  1 teaspoon molasses or sorghum
  1 tablespoon ground flaxseed
Rose hip tea

Snack 1 orange or 2 tangerines

Lunch 3 ounces herring or sardines
1 cup steamed asparagus
½ cup brown or wild rice with fresh ginger
½ cup steamed bamboo shoots
6 to 8 baked mushrooms stuffed with whole wheat bread crumbs and
  garlic
½ cup mandarin oranges
Blackberry tea

Snack 1 cup fresh popcorn

Dinner 1 glass (6 ounces) fresh grapefruit juice*
4 ounces broiled fish** or fowl*** (without skin)
Corn on cob (1 ear)
½ cup barley pearls with ½ cup mushrooms
2 slices rye bread
Salad:
  6 to 8 asparagus spears (steamed)
  ½ cup Bermuda onion slices
  ½ cup wheat sprouts
Dressing:
  1 tablespoon corn oil and ¼ lemon (juice)
½ cup tapioca (vanilla) with ½ cup fresh strawberries or raspberries

Bedtime Rose hip tea

*Juice should be freshly squeezed.
**Families: sturgeon, paddlefish, tarpon, herring, whitefish, smelt.
***Duck or goose.

FOOD FAMILIES: DAY 3

Apple   Apple, pear, quince
Mulberry   Mulberry, fig, breadfruit
Honeysuckle   Elderberry
Goosefoot (Beet)   Beet, spinach, chard, lamb's-quarters (greens), sugar beet
Mallow   Okra, cottonseed
Protea   Macadamia nut
Walnut   English walnut, black walnut, pecan, hickory nut, butternut
Mint   Basil, savory, sage, oregano, horehound, catnip, spearmint, peppermint, thyme, marjoram, lemon balm
Quail   Quail, peafowl, pheasant, chicken, chicken eggs
Sole
Ocean Perch, Rosefish
Sea Robins, Sea Tags
Puffer

Tea   Elderberry, mint
Oil   Cottonseed
Sweetener   Beet sugar, clover, sage honey (if honey was not used on another day of the rotation)
Juice   Juices (unsweetened) may be made from any of the fruits or vegetables listed above, including fresh herbs

SAMPLE DIET: DAY 3

Breakfast   1 glass (6 ounces) fresh apple juice
2 dried figs or 4 fresh figs
2 eggs, soft-boiled or poached, or omelette (without milk)
Elderberry tea
Snack   Handful (1 ounce) macadamia nuts and 1 sour apple (MacIntosh)
Lunch   1 glass (4 ounces) pear nectar
4 ounces broiled fish* or broiled fowl (quail family)**
1 cup steamed beets
1 cup steamed Swiss chard
Salad:
1 cup raw spinach
1 ounce chopped walnuts
Fresh basil leaves
Dressing:
1 tablespoon cottonseed oil and herbs (mint family)
Snack   Handful (1 ounce) pecans
1 pear or 1 Delicious apple
Dinner   1 glass (4 ounces) fresh apple juice
4 ounces quail (without skin)
1 cup baked breadfruit
1 cup steamed okra
½ cup applesauce (unsweetened)
Salad:
½ cup shredded beets
1 cup lamb's-quarters (greens) or chard
1 sliced, hard-boiled egg
Dressing:
1 tablespoon cottonseed oil and herbs (mint family)
1 pear or 1 quince (¼ cup, sweetened with beet sugar)
Bedtime   Peppermint tea

*Families: sole, ocean perch, sea robins, puffer.
**Family: quail (quail, peafowl, pheasant, chicken, chicken eggs).

FOOD FAMILIES: DAY 4

Banana   Banana, plantain, psyllium seed
Grape   Grapes (all varieties), raisins
Aster   Lettuce, chicory, endive, escarole, artichoke, Jerusalem artichoke, dandelion, sunflower seed and oil, tarragon, safflower oil, chamomile, goldenrod
Laurel   Avocado, cinnamon, bay leaf, sassafras, cassia buds or cassia bark
Conifer   Pine nuts
Grouse
Porgy
Mackerel   Atlantic mackerel, Spanish mackerel, king mackerel, bluefish tuna, bonito, frigate mackerel, skipjack tuna
Butterfish
Flounder   Flounder, halibut
Cockles
Clams
Abalone
Lobster
Crab

Tea   Chamomile, sassafras
Oil   Sunflower seed, safflower
Sweetener   Avocado honey (if honey was not used on another day of the rotation), fructose
Juice   Juices (unsweetened) may be made from any of the fruits or vegetables listed above

SAMPLE DIET: DAY 4

Breakfast 1 glass (4 ounces) grape juice
1 sliced banana
Raisin and nut cereal*
Sassafras tea with 1 teaspoon fructose
Snack ½ ripe avocado or handful (1 ounce) of sunflower seeds
Lunch 6 ounces broiled or steamed shellfish** or 4 ounces broiled grouse
(without skin)
1 cup steamed Jerusalem artichokes
Salad:
   4 artichoke hearts (globe)
   1 cup romaine or Boston lettuce
   ½ cup endive
Dressing:
   1 tablespoon sunflower seed butter or oil with tarragon
1 cup red grapes
Snack Handful (1 ounce) pine nuts
2 ounces raisins
Dinner 1 glass (4 ounces) grape juice
4 ounces broiled fish***
1 cup baked plantains
Large steamed artichoke (globe)
Salad:
   1 cup chicory
   ½ cup escarole
   Dandelion leaves
   ½ avocado
   3 or 4 sliced Jerusalem artichokes (raw)
Dressing:
   Safflower oil and tarragon
White grapes (1 cup)
Bedtime Chamomile tea

*Raisin and nut cereal: 2 ounces raisins and 2 ounces nuts (pine nuts, sunflower seeds,
psyllium seeds), ground to make a fine cereal.
**Families: cockles, clams, abalone, lobster or crab.
***Families: porgy, mackerel, butterfish, flounder.

FOOD FAMILIES: DAY 5

Heath (Blueberry)   Blueberry, huckleberry, cranberry, wintergreen
Holly   Pokeberry, bearberry
Plum   Plum, prune, cherry, peach, apricot, nectarine, almond, persimmon (ebony), wild cherry
Parsley   Carrot, parsnip, parsley, celery, celery seed, celeriac, anise, dill, fennel, cumin, coriander, caraway, chervil
Pedalium   Sesame seed, sesame paste (tahini), oil, sesame butter
Sapucaia   Brazil nut
Sweet Potato (Morning Glory) or Yam
Turkey
Swine   Pork, pork products
Fish   Grunt, yellow perch, bluefish, pompano, dolphin fish, whiting

---

Tea   Blueberry, berry, fennel
Oil   Almond oil and butter, sesame oil **and** butter, tahini (sesame paste)
Sweetener   Tupelo or wildflower honey (if not used on another day of the rotation)
Juice   Juices (unsweetened) may be made from any of the fruits or vegetables listed above

SAMPLE DIET: DAY 5

Breakfast   1 glass (4 ounces) apricot nectar
Fruit and nut cereal* with 1 teaspoon tupelo honey
1 cup fresh blueberries or cherries
Maté tea
Snack   Handful raw almonds and 1 nectarine or 2 plums
Lunch   1 glass (4 ounces) prune juice
4 ounces broiled fish**
1 cup baked sweet potato
1 cup steamed celeriac or chervil
Salad:
   ½ cup shredded carrots
   4 celery stalks
   ½ cup chopped parsley
   1 cup anise or fennel leaves
Dressing:
   1 tablespoon sesame oil and caraway seeds
½ cup stewed prunes
Snack   4 celery stalks with almond butter
Dinner   1 glass (4 ounces) peach nectar
4 ounces lean pork (broiled) or 4 ounces broiled turkey (without skin)
1 cup steamed carrots with dill
½ cup baked parsnips or yam
1 cup steamed fennel
Celery sticks, carrot curls, with 1 teaspoon sesame butter or tahini
1 ripe persimmon
Fennel tea
Bedtime   Blueberry tea

*Fruit and nut cereal: 3 ounces dried apricots, prunes (chopped) and 2 ounces nuts
(Brazil nuts, almonds; sesame seeds), ground to a fine cereal.
**Families: grunt, yellow perch, bluefish, pompano, dolphin fish, whiting.

FOOD FAMILIES: DAY 6

Pawpaw   Pawpaw, papaya, papain
Custard   Cherimoya
Cashew   Cashew, pistachio, mango
Legume   Black-eyed pea, carob (St.-John's-bread, locust bean), fava or broad bean (vetch), alfalfa, garbanzo (chick-pea), snap bean, goober, green pea, kidney bean (frijol), lentil, licorice, lima bean, mung bean, navy bean, peanut (and oil), pigeon pea, pinto bean, soybean, soy flour, lecithin, soybean oil, string bean, tamarind, wax bean, snowpea; sprouts (mung, soybean, chick-pea, lentil, alfalfa)
Cyperaceae   Chinese water chestnut
Beech   Beechnut, chestnut
Guinea fowl
Mullet
Bass   Striped bass, rockfish, spotted bass, black sea bass, grouper, hind, white perch
Black Bass   Largemouth black bass, smallmouth black bass, spotted black bass, sunfish, pumpkinseed, bluegill
Red Snapper
Shrimp
Scallops
Oysters
Snails
Squid

Tea   Papaya, licorice, alfalfa
Oil   Soybean, peanut
Sweetener   Carob syrup, alfalfa honey (if honey was not used on another day of the rotation)
Juice   Juices (unsweetened) may be made from any of the fruits or vegetables listed above, including fresh sprouts

SAMPLE DIET: DAY 6

Breakfast 1 glass (4 ounces) papaya juice
1 cup papaya, mango or cherimoya (fresh)
2 ounces raw cashews, peanuts or beechnuts
Papaya tea

Snack 1 ounce pistachios and ½ fresh papaya or pawpaw

Lunch 1 cup lentil soup
4 ounces steamed or broiled shellfish* or 4 ounces broiled guinea fowl (without skin)
1 cup black-eyed peas
Salad (any available sprouts**):
    2 cups alfalfa, mung, lentil and soy sprouts
Dressing:
    1 tablespoon fresh peanut butter***
Mango slices

Snack 6 roasted chestnuts

Dinner 1 cup pea soup
4 ounces broiled fish†
1 cup steamed green beans with ¼ cup sliced water chestnuts
½ cup lima, kidney, navy, pinto, mung or fava beans
Salad:
    1 cup alfalfa or mung sprouts with ¼ cup mashed chick-peas and 1 tablespoon soybean oil
½ cup chestnut purée (sweetened with carob syrup)
Alfalfa tea

Bedtime Licorice tea

  *Families: shrimp, scallops, oysters, snails, squid.
  **See instructions for sprouting.
***Peanut butter should be fresh, nonhydrogenated variety.
  †Families: mullet, bass, black bass, red snapper.

FOOD FAMILIES: DAY 7

Gourd   Watermelon, cantaloupe, winter melon and other melons, pumpkin,
cucumber, zucchini, squash; pumpkin and squash seeds
Gooseberry   Currant, gooseberry
Potato   Potato, tomato, eggplant, red and green pepper, chili pepper, paprika,
cayenne
Pepper   Black and white pepper, peppercorns
Myrtle   Allspice, cloves, guava, pimento
Olive   Black or green olives
Nutmeg   Nutmeg, mace
Ginseng   Ginseng root
Maple   Maple sugar and syrup
Pigeon
Northern Pike   Northern pike, muskellunge
Buffalo   Buffalo, sucker
Carp
Catfish
Cod   Cod, haddock, pollack, tomcod, silver hake
Eel   Common, conger

Tea   Ginseng
Oil   Olive
Sweetener   Maple syrup
Juice   Juices (unsweetened) may be made from any of the fruits or vegetables
listed above, including melons

SAMPLE DIET: DAY 7

Breakfast Ginseng tea
1 glass (6 ounces) melon juice*
1 whole cantaloupe or ½ larger melon (honeydew, casaba, Persian melon; or 4 inch × 4 inch wedge of watermelon)**

Snack 2 ounces pumpkin or squash seeds
1 ounce currants

Lunch 1 glass (8 ounces) fresh tomato-cucumber juice
4 ounces broiled pigeon (without skin)
1 medium baked potato
1 cup steamed zucchini
6 green olives stuffed with pimento
Salad:
   Sliced tomato
   ½ cucumber, sliced
   ½ red or green pepper, sliced
Dressing:
   1 tablespoon olive oil, paprika or cayenne pepper

Snack 1 ounce currants

Dinner 1 glass (8 ounces) fresh tomato juice
4 ounces broiled fish***
1 cup baked butternut or acorn squash with allspice
1 cup stewed zucchini, eggplant and tomato
Cucumber slices; 6 black olives
½ cantaloupe or other small melon**

Bedtime Ginseng tea

*Whole melon, including seeds, may be juiced in a blender, then strained, for nutritious drink.

**Melon should be eaten 1 to 2 hours after the meal if it produces gas when eaten immediately after the meal.

***Families: northern pike, buffalo, carp, catfish, cod, eel.

APPENDIX 3:
Tests to Determine Predisposing Factors

Laboratory tests can often be helpful in uncovering predisposing factors to a brain sensitivity. Although the specific tests ordered need to be individualized in accordance with each person's medical history and physical examination, the following is a compilation of tests we frequently order:

1. *CBC (Complete Blood Count).* A blood test measuring the number of white blood cells, the number of red blood cells, and the hemoglobin content of the red blood cells (hemoglobin is needed for oxygen transport). It is helpful in determining the presence or absence of anemia, infection, and other blood disorders.

2. *ESR (Erythrocyte Sedimentation Rate).* A blood test which measures the speed at which erythrocytes (red blood cells) settle. It is used as a screening test for tissue inflammation.

3. *Biochemical Profile.* A group of tests done from a single sample of blood, which tests a variety of important chemical components. Although the specific grouping of tests may vary somewhat from profile to profile, they generally include: Cholesterol and/or Triglycerides, which pertain to the metabolism of fat; Albumin Total Protein and Uric Acid, which pertain to the metabolism of protein; Glucose, which pertains to carbohydrate metabolism; Bilirubin; LDH; Alkaline Phosphatase; SGOT; SGPT, which, among other things, indicates how the liver is functioning; BUN and Creatinine, indicators of kidney functioning. In addition, usually these profiles also measure the blood level of the following minerals: calcium, phosphorous, chlorides, sodium and potassium.

4. *Mauve Factor.* A urine test which screens for the presence of an abnormal chemical that is capable of interfering with proper brain functioning.

5. *Twenty-Four-Hour Urine for 17 Hydroxy and 17 Keto Steroids.* The total urinary output for a twenty-four-hour period is analyzed for specific hormones, which primarily gives information about the functioning of the adrenal glands and the gonads.

6. *T-3, T-4, TSH.* Blood tests that measure the level of hormones related to the functioning of the thyroid gland. However, as indicated on pages 117–118, thyroid blood levels are not always accurate indicators of thyroid function.

There is a way to test for thyroid functioning which can be safely done at home and without expense. This test, known as the axillary temperature test, was researched extensively by Dr. Broda Barnes. (Barnes, Broda O., and Galton, Lawrence, *Hypothyroidism: The Unsuspected Illness,* published by Thomas Y. Crowell Co., Inc., New York, 1976.) The test is based on measuring an actual function of the thyroid gland—maintaining the proper basal temperature (the temperature of the body at rest). The test is carried out by taking the axillary (underarm) temperature first thing in the morning before getting out of bed. A thermometer is prepared the night before (shaken down and left at the bedside within easy reach) and, on awakening, is inserted under the armpit and held in place (by lowering the arm against the body) for ten minutes, at the end of which time the temperature is noted.

The normal temperature, when taken in this manner, ranges from 97.8° to 98.2°. Temperatures below this range may be indicative of low-thyroid functioning. It is advisable to record the temperature on at least three separate days so that variations, if present, may be noted. For women, the most accurate results are obtained if the temperatures are recorded on the first three days of the menstrual cycle (first three days of bleeding).

7. *Glucose Tolerance Test.* This blood test is primarily used to diagnose diabetes and hypoglycemia. It involves fasting for ten to twelve hours. A blood sample is then taken to determine your fasting blood sugar level. Then you are given a drink containing a measured amount of glucose. Following this, blood samples are drawn at specific intervals (half hour, one hour and hourly up to six hours) to determine what happens to your blood sugar level.

The following criteria are among those we use to diagnose hypoglycemia (these are in addition to an obvious drop in blood sugar below the normal cutoff point):

(1) A failure of the blood sugar to rise (after ingestion of the test dose of glucose) at least 50mg percent above the fasting blood sugar mark.

(2) A drop in blood sugar, at any time during the test, of 20mg percent or more below the fasting blood sugar mark.

(3) The subjective development of symptoms, at any time during the test, which correlate with a drop in blood sugar.

8. *Hair Analysis.* Approximately two tablespoonfuls of hair is cut (usually from the nape of the neck) and sent to a laboratory equipped to analyze the hair for its mineral content. Excesses and deficiencies of minerals can be determined, as well as the levels of toxic metals (such as lead and mercury).

9. *Gastro-Intestinal pH Measurement.* A relatively simple procedure that can measure the pH level of the stomach and intestines. The test involves the swallowing of a capsule (about the size used for vitamins or antibiotics) which has built into it a miniature pH meter and radio transmitter. Once swallowed, the capsule continuously transmits the pH value from the gastro-intestinal tract. The signals are picked up by an antenna (which is built into a wide belt and worn around the abdomen) and recorded on a graph similar to an electrocardiogram. The capsule leaves the body through the normal process of elimination.

This test can be used to determine: (1) the pH of the stomach (it can diagnose hyperacidity, as well as insufficient amounts of stomach acid); (2) the pH of the small intestine; and (3) the emptying time of the stomach (length of time food stays in stomach before passing into the small intestine). The pH of the small intestine can be monitored while testing individual foods. If the pH fails to go up after eating a food, this would be evidence of an allergic response which is inhibiting the pancreas.

APPENDIX 4:
Sprouting Seeds

THE WHY OF SPROUTING

Seeds have long been a part of the human diet. The seed of a plant not only contains the blueprints of what that plant can become, but is also rich in vitamins, minerals, enzymes and protein.

The process of sprouting activates the life-giving force within the seed and allows it to grow. During the first few days of growth, the concentration of vitamins and proteins increases greatly. Thus, sprouting markedly enhances the nutritional value of seeds and yields a crop of natural, tasty, fresh food—all in a matter of three to five days in the convenience of your kitchen and without much expense or work.

WHAT TO SPROUT

Almost all seeds are good for sprouting. There are some exceptions, such as tomato seeds and potato sprouts. These are considered poisonous and should be avoided. When you buy sprouting seeds, try to buy organic seeds or edible seeds that have not been raised or treated chemically. Many chemical sprays and fumigants not only inhibit or prevent sprouting but are harmful to humans. You may obtain help on this from a health food store, the new health food departments in some supermarkets, and garden supply stores. The basic rule is to avoid chemically treated seeds.

A partial list of seeds for sprouting includes: alfalfa, barley, beet, buckwheat, caraway, celery, chia, clover, corn, cress, dill, fava, fenugreek, flax, garbanzo, kale, lentil, lettuce, pinto, purslane, pumpkin, radish, rye, safflower, sesame, soy, sunflower, turnip and wheat.

HOW TO SPROUT

You can get very good results with seeds, beans or grains (or a combination of seeds or grains) by carefully following these directions:

1. Pick over the seeds carefully, retaining for sprouting only clean, whole seeds.

2. Place two to three tablespoons of the seeds in a one-quart glass jar.

3. Cover with at least three-fourths cup lukewarm water and let stand for a few hours (or, at most, overnight) until they are swollen (we suggest using spring water).

4. Pour off this water; then rinse the seeds thoroughly, making sure to pour off all excess water.

5. Cover the top of the jar with a piece of cheesecloth or sprouting wire and tie securely.

6. Place the jar on its side in a cupboard or any dark place.

7. Three times a day pour plenty of water over the seeds, carefully washing and rinsing the seeds. The more thorough the washing, the better the sprouts will be. Be sure to drain off all excess water. After washing, place the jar on its side as before.

8. In three to five days the sprouts will be developed. They should be taken out of the jar before they develop rootlets. Wash and drain, and then store in the refrigerator for use in salads, snacks, for cooking, etc.

If you desire chlorophyll in your sprouts, remove the lid from your sprouter during the final hours before harvesting and exposing to indirect sunlight.

Any sprouts not immediately used may be stored in your refrigerator in a covered container and will generally keep for three to five days. However, the sooner they are eaten, the higher will be the nourishment.

Here is a table showing the recommended lengths of the sprouts of various seeds. When the sprout reaches the approximate length shown, it should be harvested and either eaten immediately or placed in the refrigerator to inhibit further sprouting.

Buckwheat	1 to 1½ inches
Alfalfa, clover, flax	¾ to 1 inch
Radish, turnip	½ to 1 inch
Garbanzo	½ to ¾ inch
Corn, mung, pea, soybean	¼ to ½ inch

| Lentil, oat, rye, wheat | No longer than the seed |
| Sesame, sunflower, fenugreek | Barely budded |

Beware of letting sesame seed, fenugreek or sunflower seed sprout too much. They are ready to eat blended into milk and are at their sweetest when you can just barely see the sprout starting out of the seed.

APPENDIX 5:
The Kaiser
Permanente (K-P)
or Feingold Diet

The K-P diet involves eliminating the following two groups of foods:
1. Foods Containing Natural Salicylates. These foods are:

Vegetables Tomatoes and all tomato products, Cucumbers (pickles)

Nuts Almonds

Fruit Apples, Apricots, Berries—Blackberries, Boysenberries, Gooseberries, Raspberries, Strawberries—Cherries, Currants, Grapes (and grape products: e.g., wine, wine vinegar, raisins, jellies, etc.), Nectarines, Oranges (*Note:* Grapefruits, lemons and limes are permitted), Peaches, Plums, Prunes

In the diets of children who are sensitive to them, salicylates must be omitted in any and all forms—fresh, frozen, canned, dried, as juice, or as an ingredient of prepared foods.

2. Any Food Containing a Synthetic (Artificial Color or Flavor) or BHT (Butylated Hydroxy Toluene).

A wide variety of processed foods and drugs contain these substances. Labels must be read carefully.

To try this diet, eliminate all foods from groups 1 and 2 for six weeks. If the child responds well to the diet, foods from group 1 may be added one at a time every three to four days. Should the child react adversely to any of the added foods, those foods are to be eliminated indefinitely. All foods from group 2 are eliminated permanently.

APPENDIX 6:
Resource
Organizations

Professional organizations concerned with clinical ecology, nutrition, orthomolecular medicine, preventive medicine and/or kinesiology

Society for Clinical Ecology
Robert Collier, M.D., Secretary
4045 Wadsworth Blvd.
Wheat Ridge, CO 80033
Society for physicians and scientists concerned with the effects of our total environment. Maintains a list of physicians who carry out the various allergy-diagnostic procedures discussed in this book.

Academy of Orthomolecular Psychiatry
1691 Northern Blvd.
Manhasset, NY 11030
Professional organization consisting primarily of psychiatrists (but also physicians of other specialties, psychologists and scientists) interested in orthomolecular psychiatry. Maintains a referral list.

International Academy of Preventive Medicine
10409 Town and Country Way
Suite 200
Houston, TX 77024
Professional organization consisting of physicians, dentists, and other health-care practitioners concerned with preventive medicine, nutrition, kinesiology and allergies. Maintains a referral list.

American Academy of Medical Preventics
2811 "L" St.
Sacramento, CA 95816
213-878-1234
Professional organization of physicians interested in chelation therapy (as it relates to the treatment of heavy metal poisoning and degenerative diseases), nutrition and preventive medicine. Maintains a referral list.

Society for Orthomolecular Medicine
2340 Parker St.
Berkeley, CA 94704
Professional organization that sponsors scientific meetings on orthomolecular medicine.

International College of Applied Nutrition
Box 386
La Habra, CA 90631
Professional organization consisting of physicians and scientists interested in applied nutrition.

International Academy of Metabology, Inc.
1000 E. Walnut St.
Suite 247
Pasadena, CA 91106
Professional organization concerned with nutrition and ecology.

International Academy of Biological Medicine, Inc.
P.O. Box 31313
Phoenix, AZ 85404
Professional organization of health care practitioners interested in biological approach to health and disease. Maintains a referral list.

International College of Applied Kinesiology
586 Michigan Bldg. (Dr. George Goodheart)
Detroit, MI 48226
Professional organization of health care practitioners interested in applied kinesiology.

The Institute of Behavioral Kinesiology
376 F Jeffrey Pl. (John Diamond, M.D.)
Valley Cottage, NY 10989

Professional organization of health care practitioners interested in behavioral kinesiology.

Resources for information on clinical ecology, orthomolecular medicine, preventive medicine and/or nutrition

New England Foundation for Allergic and Environmental Diseases
The Alan Mandell Center for Bio-Ecologic Diseases
3 Brush St.
Norwalk, CT 06850
Distributes literature and conducts research on clinical ecology.

The Human Ecology Research Foundation
720 N. Michigan Ave.
Chicago, IL 60611
Distributes literature and supports research in clinical ecology. Articles by Dr. Theron Randolph available from this group.

The Huxley Institute
1114 First Ave.
New York, NY 10021
212-759-9554
Distributes information on orthomolecular psychiatry and medicine. Maintains referral list for physicians practicing in these fields.

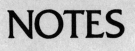

NOTES

The words following the page numbers conclude the material to which reference is made.

ONE: BRAIN SENSITIVITY AND YOU

p. 8   causing the sensitivity. Theron G. Randolph, "Descriptive Features of Food Addiction," *Quarterly J. Studies of Alcohol* 17 (1956): 198.

p. 8   cycle of sensitivity: Herbert J. Rinkel, Theron G. Randolph, and Michael Zeller, *Food Allergy* (Springfield, Ill.: Charles C Thomas, 1951), pp. 3–53.

p. 9   *masked* food sensitivities . . . *Ibid.*

p. 11 revolutionary ideas. Wayne Martin, *Medical Heroes and Heretics* (Old Greenwich, Conn.: The Devin-Adair Co., 1977).

p. 11 book *Silent Spring* . . . Rachel Carson, *Silent Spring* (Boston: Houghton Mifflin Co., 1962).

p. 11 clinical immunologists. Randolph, "Historical Development of Clinical Ecology," in Lawrence D. Dickey, *Clinical Ecology* (Springfield, Ill.: Charles C Thomas, 1976), pp. 9–17.

p. 12 allergic response. *Ibid.*

p. 15 disease present. Josef Breuer and Sigmund Freud, *Studies on Hysteria (1893–1895)*; Sigmund Freud, *The Standard Edition of the Complete Psychological Works of Sigmund Freud* (London: The Hogarth Press, 1955).

TWO: CRACKPOT THEORY OR ESTABLISHED FACT?

p. 18 custom of taking once." Francis Adams, *The Genuine Works of Hippocrates* (Baltimore: Williams & Wilkins, 1939), cited in Dickey, "History and Documentation of the Food Factors of Disease Food Allergy—Fact or Fancy?," in Dickey, *Clinical Ecology* (Springfield, Ill.: Charles C Thomas, 1976), p. 29.

p. 19 alcoholic drinks. . . ." Francis Hare, *The Food Factor in Disease*, vols. I, II (London: Longmans, 1905), cited in Dickey, *op. cit.*, p. 27.

p. 19 allergy to eggs. A. T. Schofield, "A Case of Egg Poisoning," *Lancet* 1 (1908): 716.

p. 19 functional hypoglycemia. Seale Harris, "Hyperinsulinism and Dysinsulinism," *JAMA* 83 (Sept. 6, 1924): 729–33.

p. 19 *Diagnosis and Treatment*). Albert H. Rowe, *Food Allergy: Its Manifestations, Diagnosis, and Treatment* (Philadelphia: Lea & Febiger, 1931).

p. 20 period of abstinence. Richard Mackarness, *Eating Dangerously: The Hidden Hazards of Food Allergies* (New York and London: Harcourt Brace Jovanovich, 1976), pp. 50–52.

p. 22 by teacher expectations. R. Rosenthal and L. Jacobson, "Teacher Expectancies: Determinants of Pupils' I.Q. Gains," *Psychological Reports* 19 (1966): 115–18.

p. 22 has been questioned. Abram Hoffer and Humphry Osmond, *Megavitamin Therapy: In Reply to the American Psychiatric Association Task Force on Megavitamin and Orthomolecular Therapy in Psychiatry* (Regina, Saskatchewan: Canadian Schizophrenia Foundation, 1976), pp. 80–94.

p. 23 psychiatric journals. F. C. Dohan *et al.*, "Relapsed Schizophrenics' More Rapid Improvement on a Milk-and-Cereal–Free Diet," *Br. J. Psychiatry* 115 (1969): 595–96;

F. C. Dohan and J. C. Grasberger, "Relapsed Schizophrenics' Earlier Discharge from the Hospital After Cereal-Free, Milk-Free Diet," *Am. J. Psychiatry* 130, no. 6 (June 1973): 685–88.

p. 23 Singh and Kay. Manmohan Singh and Stanley R. Kay, "Wheat Gluten as a Pathogenic Factor in Schizophrenia," *Science* (January 30, 1976): 401–2.

p. 24 book *Eating Dangerously*. Mackarness, *op. cit.*, pp. 3–27.

p. 30 Feingold and others. Ben F. Feingold, *Why Your Child Is Hyperactive* (New York: Random House, 1974); *idem*, "Hyperkinesis and Learning Disabilities Linked to Artificial Food Flavors and Colors," *Am. J. Nursing* 75 (1975): 797–803; C. K. Conners *et al.*, "Food Additives and Hyperkinesis: A Controlled Double-Blind Experiment," *Pediatrics* 58, no. 2 (1976): 154–66; Clyde Hawley and Robert E. Buckley, "Sensitivity to Food Dyes in Hyperkinetic Children," *J. Applied Nutrition* 26, no. 4 (1974): 57–61; *idem*, "Hyperkinesis and Sensitivity to the Aniline Food Dyes," *J. Orthomolecular Psychiatry* 5, no. 2 (1976): 129–37.

p. 30 containing salicylates. Feingold, *Why Your Child Is Hyperactive*.

THREE: FASTING AND DELIBERATE FOOD TESTING

p. 36 than before it." Paavo O. Airola, *Are You Confused?* (Phoenix: Health-Plus Publishers, 1971), p. 106.

p. 36 United States for years. Randolph, "An Ecologic Orientation in Medicine: Comprehensive Environmental Control in Diagnosis and Therapy," *Ann. Allergy* 23 (1965): 7; *idem*, "The Ecologic Unit," *Hospital Management* 97 (March 1964): 45; 97 (April 1964): 46.

FOUR: THE COCA PULSE TEST

p. 54 inhalants and chemicals. Arthur F. Coca, *The Pulse Test* (New York: Arco Publishing Co., 1956).

FIVE: KINESIOLOGIC TESTING

p. 63 applied kinesiology. George Goodheart, *Collected Papers* (Detroit: International College of Applied Kinesiology, 1969); David S. Walther, *Applied Kinesiology* (Pueblo, Colo.: Systems DC, 1976).

p. 69 Dr. John Diamond ... John Diamond, *Collected Papers* (Valley Cottage, N.Y.: The Institute of Behavioral Kinesiology, 1977); *idem*, *Behavioral Kinesiology* (New York: Harper & Row, 1979).

SIX: FOUR LABORATORY TESTS

p. 74 food allergies. Feingold, *Introduction to Clinical Allergy* (Springfield, Ill.: Charles C Thomas, 1973), p. 148.

p. 74 began to swell. Dickey, "History and Documentation of Coseasonal Antigen Therapy, Intracutaneous Serial Dilution Titration, Optimal Dosage and Provocative Testing," in *idem*, *Clinical Ecology* (Springfield, Ill.: Charles C Thomas, 1976), pp. 20–22.

p. 74 Rinkel's method. *Ibid.*, pp. 22, 23.

p. 75 between the injections. Joseph B. Miller, *Food Allergy: Provocative Testing and Injection Therapy* (Springfield, Ill.: Charles C Thomas, 1972).

p. 76 work with inhalants. Herbert A. Roberts, *The Principles and Art of Cure by Homeopathy: A Modern Textbook* (New Delhi, India: B. Jain Publishers, 1942).

p. 81 sublingual testing works. Marshall Mandell, "Cerebral Reactions in Allergic Patients" (Presented at the Twenty-fourth Annual Congress, American College of Allergists, Section on Neurologic Allergy, Washington, D.C., April 18, 1969) (Norwalk, Conn.: The New England Foundation for Allergic and Environmental Diseases).

p. 83 Dr. A. P. Black. Black, "A New Diagnostic Method in Allergic Disease, *Pediatrics* 17 (1956): 5.

p. 83 Dr. William Bryan William T. K. Bryan and Marion P. Bryan, "The Application of *In Vitro* Cytotoxic Reactions to Clinical Diagnosis of Food Allergy," *Laryngoscope* 70 (1960): 810; *idem*, "Cytotoxic Reactions in the Diagnosis of Food Allergy," in Dickey, *Clinical Ecology* (Springfield, Ill.: Charles C Thomas, 1976), pp. 426–33.

p. 89 or RAST— Torsten L. O. Berg and S. G. O. Johansson, "Allergy Diagnosis with the Radioallergosorbent Test," *J. Allergy & Clinical Immunology* 54, no. 4 (Oct. 1974): 209–21; Gerald J. Gleich and John W. Yunginger, "The Radioallergosorb-ent Test: Its Present Place and Likely Future in the Practice of Allergy," *Advances in Asthma and Allergy* 2, no. 2 (1975).

p. 89 late 1960s . . . L. Wide, H. Bennich, and S. G. O. Johansson, "Diagnosis of Allergy by an *In Vitro* Test for Allergen Antibodies," *Lancet* 2 (1967): 1105.

p. 89 discovered in 1966 . . . K. Ishizaka and T. Ishizaka, "Identification of Gamma E-Antibodies as a Carrier of Reaginic Activity, *J. Immunology* 99 (1967): 1187.

SEVEN: COMPLICATIONS

p. 94 *Stress of Life.* Hans Selye, *The Stress of Life* (New York: McGraw - Hill Co., 1956).

p. 96 food industry. Beatrice Trum Hunter, *Food Additives and Federal Policy: The Mirage of Safety* (New York: Charles Scribner's Sons, 1975); Ross Hume Hall, *Food for Naught: The Decline in Nutrition* (New York: Harper & Row, 1974).

p. 97 these chemicals. Randolph, *Human Ecology and Susceptibility to the Chemical Environment* (Springfield, Ill.: Charles C Thomas, 1962).

p. 101 such cases. Orion Truss, "Tissue Injury Induced by Candida Albicans: Mental Neurologic Manifestations," *J. Orthomolecular Psychiatry* 7, no. 1 (1978): 17–37.

EIGHT: TREATMENT

p. 110 vitamins C and B-6. William H. Philpott, "Ecologic,

Orthomolecular and Behavioral Contributions to Psychiatry," *J. Orthomolecular Psychiatry* 3, no. 4 (1974): 359–60.

p. 111 increase the pH. Randolph, "The Enzymatic, Acid, Hypoxia, Endocrine Concept of Allergic Inflammation," in Dickey, *Clinical Ecology*, pp. 577–96.

p. 113 work adequately . . . Horace Fletcher, *Fletcherism—What Is It?* (London: Ewart, Seymour & Co., Ltd.). Reprinted by photolithography (Milwaukee: Lee Foundation for Nutritional Research, 1960).

p. 114 sensitivities worsen . . . Philpott, "Selective Substance Reactivity in Pancreatic Insufficiency," *J. Orthomolecular Psychiatry* 7, no. 3 (1978): 181–89; *idem,* "Methods of Reversing the Stimuli-Evoked Pancreatic Insufficiencies of Chronic Degenerative Diseases," pp. 190–201.

p. 114 of your health. T. L. Cleave, *Saccharine Disease: The Master Disease of Our Time* (New Canaan, Conn.: Keats Publishing, 1975), pp. 28–43.

p. 115 forty-eight hours. G. D. Campbell and T. L. Cleave, "Diverticulosis and Diverticulitis," *British Medical J.* 3 (1968): 741.

p. 115 leave the body. O. N. Manousos, S. C. Truelove, and K. Lumsden, "Prevalence of Diverticulitis in the General Population of Oxford," *British Medical J.* 3 (1967): 760.

p. 115 other related diseases . . . Cleave, *op. cit.*, pp. 28–43.

p. 117 persist, as neurotic. Broda O. Barnes and Lawrence Galton, *Hypothyroidism: The Unsuspected Illness* (New York: Thomas Y. Crowell Co., 1976).

p. 119 vestigial organ. H. Friedman, ed., "Thymus Factors in Immunity," *Ann. N.Y. Academy of Science* 249 (1975).

p. 119 defense system. Friedman, *op. cit.*

p. 119 sensitivity reaction. John W. Tintera, "Endocrine Aspects of Ophthalmologic and Otolaryngologic Allergy" (Presented Before the 27th Anniversary Program of the American Society of Ophthalmologic and Otolaryngologic Allergy, Chicago: Oct. 25–26, 1969), in *Hypoadrenocorticism* (Adrenal Metabolic Research Society of the Hypoglycemia Foundation, 1969).

p. 120 animal's liver. Alan H. Nittler, *A New Breed of Doctor* (New York: Pyramid Publications/Harcourt Brace Jovanovich, 1972), p. 948.

p. 121 alcohol . . . Harold W. Lovell and John W. Tintera, "Hypoadrenocorticism in Alcoholism and Drug Addiction," *Geriatrics* 6, no. 1 (1951): 1–11.

p. 121 caffeine Tintera, "The Hypoadrenocortical State and Its Management," *N.Y. State J. Medicine* 55, no. 13 (1955).

p. 121 nicotine. P. T. Bohan and M. G. Berry, "Hypoglycemia and the Use of Tobacco, *GP* 8 (Nov. 1953): 63–64.

p. 122 Harris in 1924 Seale Harris, "Hyperinsulinism and Dysinsulinism," *JAMA* 83 (Sept. 6, 1924): 729–33.

p. 122 Dr. Carlton Fredericks. Carlton Fredericks and Herman Goodman, *Low Blood Sugar and You* (New York: Grosset & Dunlap, 1969).

p. 122 Dr. Paavo Airola Paavo O. Airola, *Hypoglycemia: A Better Approach* (Phoenix: Health-Plus Publishers, 1977).

p. 122 cortical extract (ACE) Tintera, "Hypoadrenocorticism: The Endocrinologic Approach to the Etiology and Treatment of Functional Hypoglycemia as a Factor in Adrenocortical Dysfunction" (Adrenal Metabolic Research Society of the Hypoglycemia Foundation, Inc., 1968).

p. 123 physical appearance. Ruth Mulvey Harmer, *Unfit for Human Consumption* (Englewood Cliffs, N.J.: Prentice-Hall, 1971).

p. 123 of other vitamins. Henry A. Schroeder, *The Trace Elements and Man* (Old Greenwich, Conn.: The Devin-Adair Co., 1973).

p. 123 calcium and protein. Wilfrid E. Shute and Harold J. Taub, *Vitamin E for the Healthy and Ailing Heart* (New York: Pyramid Publications/Harcourt Brace Jovanovich, 1969).

p. 124 of normal children. R. O. Pihl and M. Parkes, "Hair Element Content in Learning Disabled Children," *Science* 198 (Oct. 14, 1977): 204–6.

p. 124 chelation therapy . . . Bruce Halstead, *Chelation Therapy* (Loma Linda, Calif.: Life and Health Medical Group, 1976).

p. 124 as a team. Roger Williams, *Biochemical Individuality* (New York: John Wiley & Sons, 1956).

p. 125 to function normally. Leon E. Rosenberg, "Vitamin Dependent Genetic Disease," in *Medical Genetics*, eds. V. A. McKusick and R. Claiborne (New York: H. P. Press, 1973), pp. 73–79.

p. 125 niacin (vitamin B-3) Abram Hoffer, "Senility as a Form of Chronic Malnutrition," in *The Crisis in Health Care for the Aging* (Report of a National Conference Sponsored by the Huxley Institute for Biosocial Research, New York City, March 1972); *idem*, "Vitamin B-3 Dependent Child," *Schizophrenics* 3, no. 2 (1971): 107–13.

p. 125 pyridoxine (vitamin B-6). Carl C. Pfeiffer and Venelin Iliev, "Pyroluria Urinary Mauve Factor Causes Double Deficiency of B-6 and Zinc in Schizophrenics," *Federation Proceedings* 32, 276, Abs. #350.

p. 125 deteriorated drastically.) Weston A. Price, *Nutrition and Physical Degeneration* (Santa Monica: Price-Pottenger Nutrition Foundation, 1972) (Heritage Edition) (first published in 1937).

p. 126 continued to reproduce. Francis M. Pottenger, Jr., "The effect of heat-processed foods and metabolized Vitamin D milk on the dentofacial structures of experimental animals." *Am. I. Orthod. Oral Surg.* 32 (8): 467. 1946. (Reprints from Price-Pottenger Nutrition Foundation, Santa Monica, Calif.)

p. 126 are not biological Beatrice Trum Hunter, *The Great Nutrition Robbery* (New York: Charles Scribner's Sons, 1978), pp. 63–70.

p. 126 such as fluoride George L. Waldbott, *Fluoridation: The Great Dilemma* (Lawrence, Kans.: Coronado Press, 1978).

p. 129 hyperactivity in children. John N. Ott, *Health and Light: The Effects of Natural and Artificial Light on Man and Other Living Things* (Old Greenwich, Conn.: The Devin-Adair Co., 1973).

p. 130 sense of discomfort. Fred Soyka and Alan Edmonds, *The Ion Effect* (New York: E. P. Dutton & Co., 1977).

p. 130 treatment of burns Igho Kornblueh *et al.*, "Polarized Air as an Adjunct in the Treatment of Burns" (Philadelphia: Northeastern Hospital, 1959).

p. 130 respiratory conditions. Alfred P. Wehner, "Electro-Aerosol Therapy," *Am. J. Physical Medicine* 41 (1962).

BIBLIOGRAPHY

CHILDHOOD HYPERACTIVITY AND LEARNING PROBLEMS

Crook, William G. *Can Your Child Read? Is He Hyperactive?* Jackson, Tenn.: Pedicenter Press, 1975.

Feingold, Ben F. *Why Your Child Is Hyperactive.* New York: Random House, 1974.

CLINICAL ECOLOGY AND ALLERGY

Coca, Arthur F. *The Pulse Test.* New York: Arco Publishing Co., 1956.

Crook, William G. *Allergy: The Great Masquerader.* Jackson, Tenn.: Professional Books, 1973.

———. *Are You Allergic?* Jackson, Tenn.: Professional Books, 1978.

———. *Tracking Down Hidden Food Allergy.* Jackson, Tenn.: Professional Books, 1978.

———. *Your Allergic Child: A Guide to Normal Living for Allergic Adults and Children.* Jackson, Tenn.: Pedicenter Press, 1975.

———. *Your Child and Allergy.* Jackson, Tenn.: Professional Books, 1973 (rev. 1978).

Frazier, Claude A. *Coping with Food Allergy: Symptoms and Treatment.* New York: Quadrangle/The New York Times Book Co., 1974.

Gerrard, John W. *Understanding Allergies.* Springfield, Ill.: Charles C Thomas, 1973.

Golos, Natalie. *Management of Complex Allergies.* Norwalk, Conn.: New England Foundation of Allergic and Environmental Diseases, 1975.

Mackarness, Richard. *Eating Dangerously: The Hidden Hazards of Food Allergies.* New York and London: Harcourt Brace Jovanovich, 1976.

Ott, John N. *Health and Light: The Effects of Natural and Artificial Light on Man and Other Living Things.* Old Greenwich, Conn.: The Devin-Adair Co., 1973.

Soyka, Fred, and Edmonds, Alan. *The Ion Effect.* New York: E. P. Dutton & Co., 1977.

Taube, E. Louis. *Food Allergy and the Allergic Patient.* Springfield, Ill.: Charles C Thomas, 1973.

Waldbott, George L. *Health Effects of Environmental Pollutants.* St. Louis: C. V. Mosby Co., 1973.

Waldbott, George L.; Burgstahler, Albert W.; and McKinney, H. Lewis. *Fluoridation: The Great Dilemma.* Lawrence, Kans.: Coronado Press, 1978.

COOKBOOKS

Cadwallader, Sharon, and Ohr, Judi. *Whole Earth Cookbook.* Boston: Houghton Mifflin Co., 1972.

Davis, Adelle. *Let's Cook It Right.* New York: New American Library/Times Mirror Co., 1970.

Ewald, Ellen Buchman. *Recipes for a Small Planet.* New York: Ballantine Books, 1973.

Ford, Marjorie Winn; Hillyard, Susan; and Kooch, Mary Faulk. *The Deaf Smith Country Cookbook.* New York: Collier/Macmillan, 1973.

Hunter, Beatrice Trum. *The Natural Foods Cookbook.* Moonachie, N.J.: Pyramid Publications/Harcourt Brace Jovanovich, 1961 (24th printing 1976).

Kinderlehrer, Jane. *Confessions of a Sneaky Organic Cook . . . or How to Make Your Family Healthy When They're Not Looking.* Emmaus, Pa.: Rodale Press, 1971.

Roth, June. *Cooking for Your Hyperactive Child.* Chicago: Contemporary Books, 1977.

————. *The Food/Depression Connection.* Chicago: Contemporary Books, 1978.

EXERCISE

Cooper, Kenneth H. *Aerobics.* New York: Bantam Books, 1972.

Fixx, James F. *The Complete Book of Running.* New York: Random House, 1977.

Hittleman, Richard L. *Yoga for Personal Living.* New York: Warner Books, 1972.

Ichazo, Oscar. *Arica Psychocalisthenics.* New York: Simon & Schuster, 1976.

Kuntzleman, Charles T., ed. *The Physical Fitness Encyclopedia.* Emmaus, Pa.: Rodale Press, 1971.

Liu, Da. *Taoist Health Exercises.* New York: Links Books, 1974.

Lowen, Alexander, and Alexander, Leslie. *The Way to Vibrant Health.* New York: Harper & Row, 1977.

Porter, Donald. *Inner Running.* New York: Grosset & Dunlap, 1978.

Royal Canadian Air Force Exercise Plans for Physical Fitness, The. New York: Pocket Books/Simon & Schuster, 1972.

Smith, David. *The East-West Exercise Book.* New York: McGraw-Hill Co., 1976.

Williams, Melvin H. *Nutritional Aspects of Human Physical and Athletic Performance.* Springfield, Ill.: Charles C Thomas, 1976.

FASTING

Airola, Paavo O. *How to Keep Slim, Healthy and Young with Juice Fasting.* Phoenix: Health-Plus Publishers, 1971 (10th ed. 1978).

Cott, Allan. *Fasting: A Way of Life.* New York: Bantam Books 1977.

Cott, Allan, *et al. Fasting: The Ultimate Diet.* New York: Bantam Books, 1975.

FOOD ADDITIVES: INTENTIONAL AND UNINTENTIONAL

Harmer, Ruth Mulvey. *Unfit for Human Consumption.* Englewood Cliffs, N.J.: Prentice-Hall, 1971.

Hunter, Beatrice Trum. *Consumer Beware!* New York: Touchstone-Clarion/Simon & Schuster, 1972.

————. *Food Additives and Federal Policy: The Mirage of Safety.* New York: Charles Scribner's Sons, 1975.

————. *The Great Nutrition Robbery.* New York: Charles Scribner's Sons, 1978.

Jacobson, Michael F. *Eater's Digest: The Consumer's Factbook of Food Additives—Are They Safe?* Garden City, N.Y.: Anchor/Doubleday, 1972.

Turner, James S. *The Chemical Feast.* New York: Grossman, 1970.

GENERAL NUTRITION

Clark, Linda. *Know Your Nutrition.* New Canaan, Conn.: Keats Publishing, 1973.

Fredericks, Carlton. *Eating Right for You.* New York: Grosset & Dunlap, 1975.

Hall, Ross Hume. *Food for Naught: The Decline in Nutrition.* New York: Harper & Row, 1974.

Kirschmann, John D. *Nutrition Almanac.* New York: McGraw-Hill, 1975.

Lappe, Frances M. *Diet for a Small Planet.* Rev. ed. New York: Ballantine Books, 1975.

Leonard, Jon N.; Hofer, J. L.; and Pritikin, Nathan. *Live Longer Now: The First 100 Years of Your Life.* New York: Grosset & Dunlap, 1976.

Null, Gary, and Null, Steve. *The Complete Handbook of Nutrition.* New York: Dell Publishing Co., 1973.

Thurston, Emory W. *Nutrition for Tots to Teens.* Encino, Calif.: Argold Press, 1976.

HYPOGLYCEMIA AND SUGAR

Abrahamson, E. M., and Pezet, A. W. *Body, Mind and Sugar.* Moonachie, N.J.: Pyramid Publications/Harcourt Brace Jovanovich, 1971.

Airola, Paavo O. *Hypoglycemia: A Better Approach.* Phoenix: Health-Plus Publishers, 1977.

Cleave, T. L. *Saccharine Disease: The Master Disease of Our Time.* New Canaan, Conn.: Keats Publishing, 1975.

Crook, William G. *Are You Bothered by Hypoglycemia?* Jackson, Tenn.: Professional Books, 1977.

Duffy, William. *Sugar Blues.* Radnor, Pa.: Chilton Book Co., 1975.

Fredericks, Carlton, and Goodman, Herman. *Low Blood Sugar and You.* New York: Grosset & Dunlap, 1969.

Yudkin, John. *Sweet and Dangerous.* New York: Wyden Books, 1972.

KINESIOLOGY

Diamond, John. *Behavioral Kinesiology.* New York: Harper & Row, 1978.

————. *Collected Papers.* Valley Cottage, N.Y.: The Institute of Behavioral Kinesiology, 1977.

Goodheart, George. *Collected Papers.* Detroit: International College of Applied Kinesiology, 1969.

Walther, David S. *Applied Kinesiology.* Pueblo, Colo.: Systems DC, 1976.

NUTRITION AND DISEASE

Airola, Paavo O. *How to Get Well.* Phoenix: Health-Plus Publishers, 1974.

Bricklin, Mark. *The Practical Encyclopedia of Natural Healing.* Emmaus, Pa.: Rodale Press, 1976.

Cheraskin, Emanuel. *Psychodietetics.* New York: Bantam Books, 1976.

Cheraskin, E.; Ringsdorf, W. M., Jr.; and Clark, J. W. *Diet and Disease.* New Canaan, Conn.: Keats Publishing, 1977.

Davis, Adelle. *Let's Get Well.* New York: New American Library/Times Mirror Co., 1965.

Diet Related to Killer Diseases, Nutrition and Mental Health. Hearing Before the Select Committee on Nutrition and Human Needs, U.S. Senate, U.S. Government Printing Office, 1977.

"Dietary Goals for the United States." Prepared by the Staff of the Select Committee on Nutrition and Human Needs, U.S. Senate, U.S. Government Printing Office, February 1977.

Ellis, John M., and Presley, James. *Vitamin B-6: The Doctor's Report.* New York: Harper & Row, 1973.

Frank, Benjamin S. *Nucleic Acid Nutrition and Therapy.* New York: Rainstone Publishing Co., 1977.

Frank, Benjamin S., and Miele, Philip. *Dr. Frank's No-Aging Diet: Eat and Grow Younger.* New York: The Dial Press, 1978.

Fredericks, Carlton. *Psycho-Nutrition.* New York: Grosset & Dunlap, 1976.

Harper, Harold W., and Culbert, Michael L. *How You Can Beat the Killer Diseases.* New Rochelle, N.Y.: Arlington House Publishers, 1978.

Kalokerinos, Archie. *Every Second Child.* Sydney, Australia: Nelson, 1974.

Nittler, Alan H. *A New Breed of Doctor.* New York: Pyramid Publications/Harcourt Brace Jovanovich, 1972.

———. *Health Questions and Answers.* New York: Pyramid Publications/Harcourt Brace Jovanovich, 1976.

Passwater, Richard A. *Supernutrition: Megavitamin Revolution.* New York: Pocket Books/Simon & Schuster, 1976.

Price, Weston A. *Nutrition and Physical Degeneration.* Santa Monica: Price-Pottenger Nutrition Foundation, 1972.

Rosenberg, Harold, and Feldzamen, A. N. *The Book of Vitamin Therapy.* New York: Berkley Publishing Corp., 1975.

Shute, Wilfrid E. *Dr. Wilfrid E. Shute's Complete, Updated Vitamin E Book.* New Canaan, Conn.: Keats Publishing, 1975.

Stone, Irwin. *The Healing Factor: Vitamin C Against Disease.* New York: Grosset & Dunlap, 1972.

Williams, Roger J. *Nutrition Against Disease.* New York: Bantam Books, 1973.

ORTHOMOLECULAR MEDICINE AND PSYCHIATRY

Hoffer, Abram, and Osmond, Humphry. *How to Live with Schizophrenia.* Rev. ed. New York: Universe Books, 1974.

———. *Megavitamin Therapy: In Reply to the American Psychi-*

atric Association Task Force on Megavitamin and Or-thomolecular Therapy in Psychiatry. Regina, Saskatchewan: Canadian Schizophrenia Foundation, 1976.

Hoffer, Abram, and Walker, Morton. *Orthomolecular Nutrition.* New Canaan, Conn.: Keats Publishing, 1978.

Megavitamin Therapy. Alberta, Canada: Final Report of the Joint University Megavitamin Therapy Review Committee to the Minister of Social Services and Community Health, December 1976.

Newbold, Henry L. *Mega-Nutrients for Your Nerves.* New York: Wyden Books, 1975.

Pfeiffer, Carl C. *Mental and Elemental Nutrients: A Physician's Guide to Nutrition and Health Care.* New Canaan, Conn.: Keats Publishing, 1976.

————. *Zn: Zinc and Other Micro-Nutrients.* New Canaan, Conn.: Keats Publishing, 1978.

Vonnegut, Mark. *The Eden Express: A Personal Account of Schizophrenia.* New York: Praeger Publishers, 1975.

STRESS REDUCTION

Benson, Herbert, and Klipper, Miriam Z. *The Relaxation Response.* New York: Avon Books, 1976.

Denniston, Denise, and McWilliams, Peter. *The TM Book: How to Enjoy the Rest of Your Life.* Los Angeles: Price/Stern/Sloan Publishers, 1975.

Durckheim, Karlfried G. *Hara, the Vital Centre of Man.* Atlantic Highlands, N.J.: Humanities Press, 1970.

Govinda, Lama A. *Creative Meditation and Multi-Dimensional Consciousness.* Wheaton, Ill.: Quest, 1976.

Huang, Al C. *Embrace Tiger, Return to Mountain: The Essence of T'ai Chi.* Moab, Utah: Real People Press, 1973.

LeShan, Lawrence. *How to Meditate: A Guide to Self-Discovery.* Boston: Little, Brown & Co., 1974.

Liu, Da. *Ta'i Chi Chu'uan and I Ching: A Choreography of Body and Mind.* New York: Harper & Row, 1972.

Ramacharaka, Yogi. *Science of Breath.* 23rd ed. Great Britain: Lowe & Brydone, 1960.

Selye, Hans. *The Stress of Life.* New York: McGraw-Hill Co., 1956.

————. *Stress Without Distress.* Philadelphia: J. B. Lippincott Co., 1974.

Tohei, Koichi. *Aikido in Daily Life.* Tokyo: Rihugei Publishing House, 1966.

Vishnudevananda, Swami. *The Complete Illustrated Book of Yoga.* New York: Pocket Books/Simon & Schuster, 1960.

THYROID

Barnes, Broda O., and Galton, Lawrence. *Hypothyroidism: The Unsuspected Illness.* New York: Thomas Y. Crowell Co., 1976.

FOR PROFESSIONALS

Barber, Theodore X., *et al.,* eds. *Biofeedback and Self-Control: An Aldine Reader on the Regulation of Bodily Processes and Consciousness.* Chicago: Aldine Publishing Co., 1971.

Breneman, James C. *Basics of Food Allergy.* Springfield, Ill.: Charles C Thomas, 1978.

Dickey, Lawrence D. *Clinical Ecology.* Springfield, Ill.: Charles C Thomas, 1976.

Feingold, Ben F. *Introduction to Clinical Allergy.* Springfield, Ill.: Charles C Thomas, 1973.

Hawkins, David, and Pauling, Linus, eds. *Orthomolecular Psychiatry: Treatment of Schizophrenia.* San Francisco: W. H. Freeman & Co., 1973.

Hosen, Harris. *Clinical Allergy: Correlated with Provocative Tests.* Hicksville, N.Y.: Exposition Press, 1978.

Jacobson, Edmund. *Progressive Relaxation.* Chicago: University of Chicago Press, 1938.

Luthe, Wolfgang. *Autogenic Training.* New York: Grune & Stratton/Harcourt Brace Jovanovich, 1965.

Luthe, Wolfgang, and Schultz, Johannes H. *Autogenic Therapy.* New York: Grune & Stratton/Harcourt Brace Jovanovich, 1959.

Miller, Joseph B. *Food Allergy: Provocative Testing and Injection Therapy.* Springfield, Ill.: Charles C Thomas, 1972.

Randolph, Theron G. *Human Ecology and Susceptibility to the Chemical Environment.* Springfield, Ill.: Charles C Thomas, 1962.

Rinkel, Herbert J.; Randolph, Theron G.; and Zeller, Michael. *Food Allergy.* Springfield, Ill.: Charles C Thomas, 1951.

Rowe, Albert H., and Rowe, Albert, Jr. *Food Allergy, Its Manifestations and Control, and the Elimination Diets—A Compendium.* Springfield, Ill.: Charles C Thomas, 1972.

Schroeder, Henry A. *The Trace Elements and Man.* Old Greenwich, Conn.: The Devin-Adair Co., 1973.

Williams, Roger J. *Physicians' Handbook of Nutritional Science.* Springfield, Ill.: Charles C Thomas, 1975.

Williams, Roger J., and Kalita, Dwight K. *A Physicians' Handbook on Orthomolecular Medicine.* Elmsford, N.Y.: Pergamon Press, 1977.

INDEX

Academy of Orthomolecular
    Psychiatry, 173
Acidity, 111, 113, 168
    See also pH level of body
Acidophilus, 115
Adaptation, 95
Addiction, 8
Additives, artificial, 30, 125,
    172
    deliberate testing of, 46
    testing for brain
        sensitivity and, 96–97
    See also specific additives
Adrenal cortical extract
    (ACE), 122
Adrenal glands, 119
Airola, Paavo, 122
Alcohol, hypoglycemia and,
    121
Allergies, 7
    See also Brain sensitivity;
        Food sensitivities
Aly, Karl-Otto, 35–36
American Academy of

    Medical Preventics, 174
Amino acids, 114
Antacids, 113
Antibodies, 89
Antigen-antibody reaction,
    83–88
Autogenic training, 129

Barnes, Broda, 167
Bentonite, 115
Biochemical profile, 166
Bioenergetic exercise, 129
Biofeedback training,
    128–29
Birds, 142
Black, A. P., 83
Blocking reactions, 110–11
Blood count, complete, 166
Blood sugar, low, see
    Hypoglycemia
Body odors, fasting and, 41
Body temperature, 167
Bowel movements, fasting
    and, 41

Brain sensitivity, 1–33
  addiction and, 8–9
  allergies and, 7–8
  chemical interference
    with testing for,
    96–100
  to chemicals, see
    Chemicals
  clinical experience with,
    25–30
  combination, 93–94
  controversy over, 10–14
  cross-sensitivities, 107
  double-blind studies of,
    21–25
  limitations of tests for,
    102
  major versus minor, 102
  as mimics, 14
  origins of concept of,
    14–17
  personal experiences with,
    31–32
  signs and symptoms of,
    135–38
  stress and thresholds of,
    94–96
  symptoms not due to,
    102–03
  symptoms of, see
    Symptoms of brain
    sensitivity
  temporary loss of, 101–
    02
  tests of, see Coca pulse
    test; Food testing,
    deliberate; Kinesiologic
    testing; Laboratory tests
  treatment of, see
    Treatment of brain
    sensitivity
  vicious cycle of, 8–9
  See also Food
    sensitivities; and specific
    topics
Breast feeding, 127
Breath, fasting and, 41
Breathing techniques, 128
Bryan, William, 83

Caffeine, hypoglycemia and,
  121
Calories in rotation diet
  menus, 140
Candles, fumes from, 27–28
Candy, 30
Carson, Rachel, 11
Chelation therapy, 124
Chemical interference,
  testing for brain
  sensitivity and, 96–100
Chemicals, 26–27, 33, 93
  in clothing, 97–98
  kinesiologic testing of, 64
  pulse testing for, 59–60
  See also Additives,
    artificial; Preservatives
Chewing food, 112–13
Children, hyperactive
  behavior in, 29–30
"Chinese restaurant
  syndrome," 32
Chocolate, 13–14
Cigarette smoking, see
  Smoking
Clinical experience with
  brain sensitivity, 25–30
Clothing
  chemicals in, 97–98
  kinesiologic testing of, 70

Coca, Arthur, 54–57
Coca pulse test, 53–61,
  90–91
  advantages and
    disadvantages of, 61
  interpreting the, 60
  preparing for, 57–58
  taking the, 58–60
  taking your pulse, 56–57
Coffee, 121
Colon, 114–15
Combination sensitivities,
  93–94
Complete blood count
  (CBC), 166
Constipation, 114, 115
Cooking, 126
Corn, 45, 49
Cross-sensitivities, 107
Crustaceans, 140–41
Cytotoxic testing, 83–88,
  90–91

Dairy products, 23–24, 142
  deliberate testing of, 45
Deliberate food testing, see
  Food testing, deliberate
Dependency, vitamin,
  124–25
Depression, 3–5, 27–28
Detoxification, fasting and,
  40–42
Diamond, John, 69
Diet(s)
  elimination, 105–06
  fats in, 126
  Kaiser Permanente (K-P)
    or Feingold, 172
  rotation, see Rotation diet
  See also Nutrition

Digestive disorders, 112–15
Digestive enzymes, 113–14
Dizziness, 12–14
Dohan, F. C., 22–23
Double-blind studies, 21–25

Ecological factors, 129–31
Ecology, clinical
  immunology versus
  clinical, 11–12
Eggs, 19–20
Electricity in the air, 130
Elimination diets, 105–06
Elimination testing, 49–52,
  90–91
Emotional factors, 103
Endocrine system, 115
  See also Hormonal
  disorders
Enemas, 41
Energy flow, kinesiologic
  testing and concept of,
  67–69
Enzymes, digestive, 113–14
Epilepsy, 55–56
Erythrocyte sedimentation
  rate (ESR), 166
Exercise, 122, 127–28
  bioenergetic, 129
  fasting and, 41
Exhaustion (fatigue), 9–10,
  26, 95

Fabrics, kinesiologic testing
  of, 70
Fast marches, Swedish,
  35–36
Fasting, 5, 9, 34–44, 51–52,
  90–91
  advantages and

disadvantages of, 51–52
benefits of, 35, 36
breaking the, 48
clues provided by, 43–44
contraindications for, 36–37
deliberate food testing without, 49–52
discomforts of, 41–43
hunger pangs and, 39–40
increased sensitivity after, 47–48
keeping a journal during, 38–39
phase one of, 39–40
phase two of, 40–43
phase three of, 43
preparing for, 37–38
Fatigue, 9–10, 26, 95
Fats in diet, 126
Feingold, Ben, 30
Feingold diet (Kaiser Permanente (K-P) diet), 172
Fertilizers, 125
Fish, 140–42
Food families, 139–42
Food sensitivities (or allergies), 19
fixed versus cyclic, 12
hidden or masked, 9, 20
See also Brain sensitivity; and specific foods
Food testing, deliberate, 33, 39, 44–52, 90–91
advantages and disadvantages of, 51–52
by elimination, 49–52
preparation for, 44–45

principles of, 45–47
without fasting (elimination testing), 49–52
Fredericks, Carlton, 122
Freud, Sigmund, 15
Fruits, 140
dried, 142
See also Juices
Fungi, 100–01

Gastro-intestinal pH measurement, 168
Glucose tolerance test, 167–68
Gluten, 23–24
Gonadal glands, 119–20
Goodheart, George, 63
Grains, 143
Grassberger, J. C., 22–23

Hair analysis, 168
Hare, Francis, 19
Harris, Seale, 19, 122
Headaches, 19
Herbs, 140
Hippocrates, 18
Honey, 142
Hormonal disorders, 115–22
hypoglycemia and, 120–22
thymus gland, 118–19
thyroid gland, 115–18
Human Ecology Research Foundation, The, 175
Hunger pangs, fasting and, 39–40
Hutton, Richard, 28–29
Huxley Institute, The, 175
Hydrochloric acid, 113

Hyperactive behavior, 29–30
Hypnotic techniques, 128
Hypoglycemia, 4, 19,
    120–22
  glucose tolerance test for,
    167–68
Hypothyroidism, 116–18

Immunoglobulins, 89
Immunology, clinical
    ecology versus clinical,
    11–12
Indigestion, 113
Inhalants, 33, 93
  kinesiologic testing, 64
  pulse taking, 59–60
  See also Smoking
Institute of Behavioral
    Kinesiology, The, 174
Insulin, hypoglycemia and,
    120–21
International Academy of
    Biological Medicine,
    Inc., 174
International Academy of
    Metabology, Inc., 174
International Academy of
    Preventive Medicine,
    173
International College of
    Applied Kinesiology,
    174
International College of
    Applied Nutrition, 174
Intestine
  large, 114–15
  small, 113–14, 168
Intradermal provocative
    testing, 73–79, 90–91

advantages and
    disadvantages of, 78–79
  neutralizing dose and,
    75–77
Ions, 130
Irritation, 20

Jewelry, kinesiologic testing
    of, 70
Juices
  fasting and, 42
  fresh, 143

Kaiser Permanente (K-P)
    diet (Feingold diet),
    172
Kay, Stanley R., 23–24
Kinesiologic testing, 62–72,
    90–91
  advantages and
    disadvantages of, 71–72
  energy flow concept and,
    67–69
  neurovascular hypothesis
    of, 66–67
  reflex hypothesis of,
    65–66
Kool-Aid, 23

Laboratory tests, 73–91
  cytotoxic testing, 83–88,
    90–91
  intradermal provocative
    testing, 73–79, 90–91
  for predisposing factors,
    166–68
  radio-allergo-sorbant test
    (RAST), 88–91
  sublingual provocative

testing, 79–83, 90–91
Large intestine, 114–15
Lee, Carleton, 74–76
Legumes, 143
Life energy, kinesiologic
   testing and concept of,
   67–69
Light (lighting), 129–30
   kinesiologic testing of, 70
Listlessness, 28–29

Mackarness, Richard, 24–25
Mandell, Marshall, 80–81
Martial arts training, 129
Mauve factor, 167
Medical lag time, 10–11
Meditation, 128
Migraines, 19
Milk, 45, 49
   breast, 127
   depression and, 4, 5
   See also Dairy products
Miller, Joseph, 75–77
Mimics, brain sensitivities
   as, 14
Minerals, 124
Mollusks, 140–41
Monosodium glutamate
   (MSG), 32
Muscles, kinesiologic testing
   of, see Kinesiologic
   testing
Music, kinesiologic testing
   of, 69

Nectars, 143
Negative ions, 130
Nervous system, 115
Neurolingual reflex, 65–66

Neurovascular hypothesis of
   kinesiologic testing,
   66–67
Neutralizing dose
   intradermal provocative
   testing and, 75–77
   therapeutic use of, 109
New England Foundation
   for Allergic and
   Environmental
   Diseases, 175
Niacin (vitamin B-3),
   dependency on, 125
Nicotine, see Smoking
Nightmares, 2–3
Nut butters, 142
Nutrition, 122–27
Nutritional supplements,
   124, 126–27
   hypoglycemia and, 122
Nuts, 126, 142

Odors, body, 41
Oils, 142
Orthomolecular psychiatry,
   4
Ott, John, 129

Pancreas, 113–14
pH level of body, 111
   gastro-intestinal
      measurement of, 168
Phlebitis, 16
Placebo effect, 21–22
Poetry, kinesiologic testing
   of, 70
Potassium bicarbonate, 114
   blocking reactions with,
   111

Poultry, 142
Predisposing factors, tests to determine, 166–68
Predisposing factors, treatment of, 112–32
  digestive disorders, 112–15
  ecological factors, 129–31
  exercise and, 122, 127–28
  hormonal disorders, *see* Hormonal disorders
  nutrition and, 122–27
  stress reduction, 122, 128–29
Preservatives, 96, 125
Price, Weston, 125
Processed foods, 123–25
Prose, kinesiologic testing of, 70
Psychoanalysis, 15–16
Psychocalisthenic programs, 129
Pulse test, Coca, 53–61, 90–91
  advantages and disadvantages of, 61
  interpreting, 60
  preparing for, 57–58
  taking, 58–60
  taking your pulse, 56–57
Pyridoxine, *see* Vitamin B-6

Radio-allergo-sorbant test (RAST), 88–91
Randolph, Theron, 20
Reflex hypothesis of kinesiologic testing, 65–66
Relaxation exercises, progressive, 128
Resource organizations, 173–75
Rinkel, Herbert, 19–20, 74
Rinkel dilution titration technique, 74
Rotation diet, 106–09
  food families and, 139–42
  four-day, 144–51
  seven-day, 152–65
Rowe, Albert, 19

Salicylates, 172
Schizophrenia, 37
Schizophrenics, double-blind studies with, 23–24
Schofield, Dr., 19
Scratch tests, 73–74
Seed butters, 143
Seeds, 126, 142
  sprouting, 169–71
Seizures, 55–56
Selye, Hans, 94
Sex glands, 119–20
Showering, fasting and, 41
Singh, Manmohan, 23–24
Skin, fasting and, 41
Sleepiness, feeling of, 9–10, 20, 47–48
Small intestine, 113–14, 168
Smoking
  deliberate testing of, 46
  hypoglycemia and, 121
  as interference in testing, 98–100
  pulse test and, 57
Snack foods, pulse test and, 57

Society for Clinical Ecology, 173

Society for Orthomolecular Medicine, 174

Sodium bicarbonate, 114
  blocking reactions with, 111

Soviet Union, 35

Soy products, 143

Spiritual essence, 131

Sprouting seeds, 169–71

Sprouts, 142

Starvation, 35

Stomach
  acidity of, 113, 168
  emptying time of, 113, 168

Stress, sensitivity thresholds and, 94–96

Stress reduction, 122, 128–29

Sublingual provocative testing, 79–83, 90–91

Sugar (refined)
  hypoglycemia and, 4, 120–21
  sleepiness and, 10
  See also Candy

Sunlight, 129–30

Swedish fast marches, 35–36

Symptoms of brain sensitivity, 6, 14, 134–38
  fasting and, 40

Symptoms of toxicity, fasting and, 40

Symptoms of withdrawal, 8

  fasting and, 40–42

Syphilis, 14

Tai-Chi, 127–28

Television, kinesiologic testing of, 69–70

Temperature, 130–31
  body, 167

Tests of brain sensitivity, see Coca pulse test; Food testing, deliberate; Kinesiologic testing; Laboratory tests

Thoughts, kinesiologic testing of, 70

Thymus gland, 118–19

Thyroid gland, 115–18
  tests of functioning of, 167

Tobacco, see Smoking

Toothpaste, 41

Toxins
  colon and, 114, 115
  fasting and, 40–41

Treatment of brain sensitivity, 104–32
  basic approaches to, 105
  blocking reactions, 110–11
  elimination diets, 105–06
  neutralizing reactions, 109
  predisposing factors, see Predisposing factors, treatment of
  rotation diets, 106–09

Twenty-four-hour urine for 17 hydroxy and 17 keto steroids, 167

Vegetables, 140
Vertigo, 12–14
Vitamin B complex, thyroid
  hormone and, 118
Vitamin B-3 (niacin),
  dependency on, 125
Vitamin B-6, 41, 95, 123
  blocking reactions with,
    110–11
  dependency on, 125
Vitamin C, 41, 95
  blocking reactions with,
    110–11
  synthetic, 127
  thyroid hormone and, 118
Vitamin dependency,
  124–25

Vitamin E, 123, 127
Vitamins, sensitivities to,
  127
Voices, kinesiologic testing
  of, 69

Water, 126
  diagnostic fast and,
    37–38, 41
Wheat, 45, 49
Wheat gluten, 23–24
Withdrawal symptoms, 8
  fasting and, 40–42

Yoga, 127
Yogurt, 115